303
Current Topics in Microbiology and Immunology

Editors

R.W. Compans, Atlanta/Georgia
M.D. Cooper, Birmingham/Alabama
T. Honjo, Kyoto · H. Koprowski, Philadelphia/Pennsylvania
F. Melchers, Basel · M.B.A. Oldstone, La Jolla/California
S. Olsnes, Oslo · M. Potter, Bethesda/Maryland
P.K. Vogt, La Jolla/California · H. Wagner, Munich

T. E. Lane (Ed.)

Chemokines and Viral Infection

With 14 Figures and 7 Tables

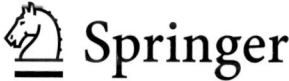

Thomas E. Lane, Ph.D.
Associate Professor
Department of Molecular Biology and Biochemistry
Center for Immunology
3205 McGaugh Hall
University of California, Irvine
Irvine, CA 92697-3900
USA
e-mail: tlane@uci.edu

Cover Illustration by Thomas E. Lane (this volume)
Chemokines and MHV-induced demyelination (see Fig. 2 of the first chapter)

Library of Congress Catalog Number 72-152360

ISSN 0070-217X
ISBN-10 3-540-29207-1 Springer Berlin Heidelberg New York
ISBN-13 978-3-540-29207-4 Springer Berlin Heidelberg New York

This work is subject to copyright. All rights reserved, whether the whole or part of the material is concerned, specifically the rights of translation, reprinting, reuse of illustrations, recitation, broadcasting, reproduction on microfilm or in any other way, and storage in data banks. Duplication of this publication or parts thereof is permitted only under the provisions of the German Copyright Law of September, 9, 1965, in its current version, and permission for use must always be obtained from Springer-Verlag. Violations are liable for prosecution under the German Copyright Law.

Springer is a part of Springer Science+Business Media
springeronline.com
© Springer-Verlag Berlin Heidelberg 2006
Printed in Germany

The use of general descriptive names, registered names, trademarks, etc. in this publication does not imply, even in the absence of a specific statement, that such names are exempt from the relevant protective laws and regulations and therefore free for general use.
Product liability: The publisher cannot guarantee the accuracy of any information about dosage and application contained in this book. In every individual case the user must check such information by consulting the relevant literature.

Editor: Simon Rallison, Heidelberg
Desk editor: Anne Clauss, Heidelberg
Production editor: Nadja Kroke, Leipzig
Cover design: design & production GmbH, Heidelberg
Typesetting: LE-TEX Jelonek, Schmidt & Vöckler GbR, Leipzig
Printed on acid-free paper   SPIN 11559986   27/3150/YL – 5 4 3 2 1 0

Preface

Chemokines represent a family of over 40 small proteins that, for the most part, are secreted into the environment and function by binding to G protein-coupled receptors (GPCRs) that are expressed on numerous different cell types. When initially identified close to 30 years ago, these molecules were associated with various human inflammatory diseases and it was recognized that expression might be integral in leukocyte recruitment to inflamed tissue [1–3]. Within a relatively short period of time, early participants within the field determined that these proteins displayed distinct and conserved structural features and exerted potent chemotactic effects on defined lymphocyte subsets [4]. There are now four subfamilies of chemokines identified based on defined structural criteria relating to the positional location of conserved cysteine residues within the amino-terminus of the protein [4, 5]. Chemokines are now recognized as important in numerous biological processes ranging from maintaining the organizational integrity of secondary lymphoid tissue to participating in various aspects of both innate and adaptive immune responses following microbial infection [6, 7].

The host response to viral infection represents a well-orchestrated ballet consisting of numerous participants with diverse roles in defense but with the ultimate goal of generating virus-specific lymphocytes whose job is to control and eliminate the invading viral pathogen from infected tissues. Over the years, an emerging picture has developed that indicates that chemokines and their receptors are intimately involved in development of effective host responses to viral pathogens. Chemokine expression is now associated with all facets of defense against viral infection including linking innate and adaptive immune responses. Early chemokine expression in response to certain viruses such as murine cytomegalovirus (MCMV) is critical in recruiting into the liver natural killer (NK) cells that control viral replication [8]. Expression of chemokines following viral infection has also been demonstrated in tissues originally thought to be relatively immunologically inert such as the central nervous system (CNS). For example, infection of the CNS with either herpes simplex virus1 (HSV-1) or mouse hepatitis virus

(MHV) results in an orchestrated expression of chemokines whose function is to attract antigen-educated lymphocytes into the CNS that contribute to the control of viral replication [9, 10]. Paradoxically, chronic expression of certain chemokines during viral persistence in CNS tissue is also associated with immune-mediated pathology [11–13]. In the face of such a robust and effective immune response, viruses have evolved various ways to avoid or distract the immune response thus enabling the establishment of infection. Certain viruses have exploited the chemokine system to their benefit by either using specific chemokine receptors as coreceptors for efficient entry into host cells (HIV) to encoding receptors with homology to chemokine receptors (various herpes and poxviruses) that may function to subvert the immune system [14–17].

Clearly, the biological roles of chemokines in host defense and/or disease are constantly evolving. This volume of *Current Topics in Microbiology and Immunology* provides an opportunity to examine the relationship between chemokines and viruses with regards to host defense and disease. In addition, the potential of chemokines and their receptors as therapeutic targets for treatment and/or prevention of disease in response to viral infection is not overlooked.

Irvine, California, July 2005   *Thomas E. Lane*

References

1. Deuel TF, Keim PS, Farmer M, Henrikson RL (1977) Amino acid sequence of human platelet factor 4. Proc Natl Acad Sci USA 74:2256
2. Luster AD, Unkeless JC, Ravetch JV (1985) Gamma-interferon transcriptionally regulates an early-response gene containing homology to platelet proteins. Nature 315:672
3. Kaplan G, Luster AD, Hancock G (1987) The expression of a gamma interferon-induced protein (IP-10) in delayed immune responses in human skin. J Exp Med 166:1098
4. Baggiolini M, Dewald B, Moser B (1994) Interleukin-8 and related chemotactic cytokines—CXC and CC chemokines. Adv Immunol 55:97
5. Luster AD (1998) Chemokines—chemotactic cytokines that mediate inflammation. N Engl J Med 338:436
6. Cyster JG (2005) Chemokines, sphingosine-1 phosphate, and cell migration in secondary lymphoid organs. Annu Rev Immunol 23:127
7. Luster AD (2002) The role of chemokines in linking innate and adaptive immunity. Curr Opin Immunol 14:129

8. Salazar-Mather TP, Orange JS, Biron CA (1998) Early murine cytomegalovirus (MCMV) infection induces liver natural killer (NK) cell inflammation and protection through macrophage inflammatory protein 1 alpha (MIP-1 alpha)-dependent pathways. J Exp Med 187:1
9. Wickham S, Lu B, Ash J, Carr DJ (2005) Chemokine receptor deficiency is associated with increased chemokine expression in the peripheral and central nervous systems and increased resistance to herpetic encephalitis. J Neuroimmunol 162:51
10. Liu MT, Chen BP, Oertel P, Buchmeier MJ, Armstrong D, Hamilton TA, Lane TE (2000) The T cell chemoattractant IFN-inducible protein 10 (IP-10) is essential in host defense against viral-induced neurologic disease. J Immunol 165:2327
11. Peterson K, Errett JS, Wei T, Dimcheff DE, Ransohoff R, Kuziel WA, Evans L, Chesebro B (2004) MCP-1 and CCR2 contribute to non-lymphocyte-mediated brain disease by Fr98 polytropic retrovirus infection in mice: role for astrocytes in retroviral neuropathogenesis. J Virol 78:6449
12. Liu MT, Keirstead HS, Lane TE (2001) Neutralization of the chemokine CXCL10 reduces inflammatory cell invasion and demyelination and improves neurological function in a viral model of multiple sclerosis. J Immunol 167:4091–4097
13. Carr DJJ, Chodosh J, Ash J, Lane TE (2003) Effect of anti-CXCL10 monoclonal antibody on HSV-1 keratitis and retinal infection. J Virol 77:10037
14. Rucker J, Doms RW (1998) Chemokine receptors as HIV coreceptors: implications and interactions. AIDS Res Hum Retroviruses 14 Suppl 3:S241
15. Alkhatib G, Combadiere C, Broder CC, Feng Y, Kennedy PE, Murhpy PM, Berger EA (1996) CC CKR5: a RANTES, MIP-1alpha, MIP-1beta receptor as a fusion cofactor for macrophage-tropic HIV-1. Science 272:1955
16. Feng Y, Broder CC, Kennedy PE, Berger EA (1996) HIV-1 entry cofactor: functional cDNA cloning of a seven transmembrane, G protein-coupled receptor. Science 272:872
17. Casarosa P, Bakker RA, Verzijl D, Navis M, Timmerman H, Leurs R, Smit MJ (2001) Constitutive signaling of the human cytomegalovirus-encoded chemokine receptor US28. J Biol Chem 276:1133

List of Contents

Functional Diversity of Chemokines and Chemokine Receptors
in Response to Viral Infection of the Central Nervous System   1
    T. E. Lane, J. L. Hardison, and K. B. Walsh

Cytokine and Chemokine Networks: Pathways to Antiviral Defense 29
    T. P. Salazar-Mather and K. L. Hokeness

Herpes Simplex Virus and the Chemokines That Mediate the Inflammation 47
    D. J. J. Carr and L. Tomanek

Influence of Proinflammatory Cytokines and Chemokines
on the Neuropathogenesis of Oncornavirus
and Immunosuppressive Lentivirus Infections 67
    K. E. Peterson and B. Chesebro

HIV-1 Coreceptors and Their Inhibitors 97
    N. Ray and R. W. Doms

A Viral Conspiracy: Hijacking the Chemokine System
Through Virally Encoded Pirated Chemokine Receptors 121
    H. F. Vischer, C. Vink, and M. J. Smit

Subject Index 155

List of Contributors

(Addresses stated at the beginning of respective chapters)

Carr, D. J. J.   47
Chesebro, B.   67

Doms, R. W.   97

Hardison, J. L.   1
Hokeness, K. L.   29

Lane, T. E.   1

Peterson, K. E.   67

Ray, N.   97

Salazar-Mather, T. P.   29
Smit, M. J.   121

Tomanek, L.   47

Vink, C.   121
Vischer, H. F.   121

Walsh, K. B.   1

Functional Diversity of Chemokines and Chemokine Receptors in Response to Viral Infection of the Central Nervous System

T. E. Lane (✉) · J. L. Hardison · K. B. Walsh

Department of Molecular Biology and Biochemistry, University of California, 3205 McGaugh Hall, Irvine, CA 92697-3900, USA
tlane@uci.edu

1	Introduction	2
1.1	Biology and Biochemistry of *Coronaviridae*	2
1.2	Immunity to MHV Infection	3
1.3	Viral Persistence and Immune-Mediated Demyelination	4
1.4	Chemokines and Chemokine Receptors	5
2	Orchestrated Expression of Chemokines and Chemokine Receptors Within the CNS Following Infection with MHV	6
3	Chemokines, Innate Immune Response, and MHV-Infection of the CNS	8
4	Chemokines and Chemokine Receptors and Their Role in Acute Viral-Induced Encephalomyelitis	9
4.1	CCL3	9
4.2	CXCL9 and CXCL10	10
4.3	CCL5	11
4.4	CCR5	11
4.5	CCL2 and CCR2	13
5	Chemokines and Chronic Viral-Induced Demyelination	14
6	Perspectives	17
	References	20

Abstract Encounters with neurotropic viruses result in varied outcomes ranging from encephalitis, paralytic poliomyelitis or other serious consequences to relatively benign infection. One of the principal factors that control the outcome of infection is the localized tissue response and subsequent immune response directed against the invading toxic agent. It is the role of the immune system to contain and control the spread of virus infection in the central nervous system (CNS), and paradoxically, this response may also be pathologic. Chemokines are potent proinflammatory molecules whose expression within virally infected tissues is often associated with protection and/or pathology which correlates with migration and accumulation of immune cells. Indeed, studies with a neurotropic murine coronavirus, mouse hepatitis virus (MHV), have provided important insight into the functional roles of chemokines and chemokine receptors in participating in various aspects of host defense as well as disease development within the CNS. This chapter will highlight recent discoveries that have provided insight into the diverse biologic roles of chemokines and their receptors in coordinating immune responses following viral infection of the CNS.

1
Introduction

1.1
Biology and Biochemistry of *Coronaviridae*

Coronaviruses are classified on the basis of several fundamental characteristics, including nucleic acid type, a lipid envelope, and their distinctive morphology [42, 64, 79]. All members have characteristic petal-shaped proteins extending from the virion surface. Coronaviruses infect numerous vertebrate hosts including humans, chickens, pigs, and mice, causing a wide variety of disorders involving a number of different organ systems; however, there are specific tropisms for the CNS, lungs, gastrointestinal tract, and liver [42, 64, 79]. Receptor use among the varied coronaviruses is restricted to several well-defined proteins. Human coronavirus infections result in acute enteritis as well as 15% of common colds indistinguishable from those caused by other viruses [42, 64, 79]. More recently, a human coronavirus has been indicated to be the etiologic agent for severe acute respiratory syndrome (SARS). SARS is a potentially lethal disease and is recognized as a health threat internationally [43].

The first murine coronavirus strain (mouse hepatitis virus, MHV), was isolated in 1949 [12]. MHV is a pathogen of wild mice, and natural infection is due to horizontal transmission, resulting in acute hepatitis with death in young animals and a variable course of persistent gastrointestinal tract infection in adults [79]. MHV is not an endemic mouse virus, but infects mouse colonies sporadically. It is very closely related to some human coronaviruses both at the genomic and protein levels. For example, human sera often contain antibody reactive to MHV. Therefore, characterizing the immune response to murine coronaviruses may provide important insight to mechanisms of control and elimination which may have important implications with regards to understanding the immune response to human coronaviruses such as the SARS coronavirus.

Coronavirus genomes are single-stranded positive-polarity RNA molecules, larger than the size of any other known stable RNA, ranging from 27 kb for the avian infectious bronchitis virus, to 31 kb for murine coronaviruses [50]. Genomic RNA is infectious, contains a cap structure at the 5′-end and poly(A) at the 3′-end. The genome is organized into seven or eight genes, each containing one or more open reading frames (ORF) separated by intergenic sequences that contain the signals for the initiation of transcription of the subgenomic viral messenger (m)RNA species. Upon entry, the viral RNA encodes an RNA polymerase that transcribes the genome into a negative-stranded RNA [50]. The latter serves as templates for positive-sensed genomic RNA and subgenomic mRNAs. Important viral structural proteins include the envelope glycoproteins (S) that bind to receptors on cell membranes [42, 64, 79]. Analysis of monoclonal antibody neutralization escape variants demonstrated that the viral S protein controls cellular tropism in vivo and the role of the S protein in tropism has recently been confirmed using stable recombinant viruses in which all genes except the S protein gene were held constant [9, 82].

1.2
Immunity to MHV Infection

The protective immune response to MHV infection is characterized predominantly by cell-mediated immunity during acute infection. A number of unique aspects of CNS viral infection have been described by analysis of the interactions between MHV and the immune response. Antibody, although protective if administered prior to infection, is not present in the serum of infected mice until after the vast majority of virus has been cleared from the CNS [56, 84]. Following infection, neutrophils, macrophages, and NK cells are rapidly recruited into the CNS, followed by T cells and B cells [104]. Inflammation is accompanied by a progressive loss of blood–brain barrier (BBB) integrity that is apparent as early as 4 days post-infection. The initial influx of innate effectors is important in facilitating T cell infiltration, as well as regulating viral replication [104]. However, the ability to survive MHV infection appears to be predominantly due to an effective T cell-mediated response [103]. Recent data have confirmed that cell-mediated immunity is critical during acute infection [53, 55, 74, 76, 92]; however, the ability to prevent viral recrudescence is associated with the continued presence of plasma cells in the CNS secreting neutralizing antibody [56, 84].

The major effectors of anti-viral immunity are virus-specific $CD8^+$ T cells. Cytotoxic T lymphocyte (CTL) induction following MHV infection of the CNS has been shown to require $CD4^+$ T cell help [92]. Although the precise mechanism or mechanisms by which $CD4^+$ T cells assist $CD8^+$ T cells have yet to be completely determined, recent studies have demonstrated that $CD4^+$ T cells are important in preventing apoptosis of CTL entering the CNS parenchyma [92]. In addition, the quality of the CTL response is $CD4^+$ T cell-dependent [92]. An important concept derived from analysis of MHV infection is that although $CD8^+$ T cells are the most prominent effectors for viral clearance during the acute infection, the mechanisms which control virus replication differ with the type of CNS cell infected. Cytolysis is important for the control of viral replication in microglia/macrophages and astrocytes while interferon (IFN)-γ is the critical effector responsible for control of virus replication in oligodendroglia [73]. The demonstration that $CD8^+$ CTL suppresses viral replication by two separate effector mechanisms, which function within the CNS in a cell type-specific manner, is an important new concept.

1.3
Viral Persistence and Immune-Mediated Demyelination

Viral persistence in white matter tracts results in a chronic demyelinating disease in which foci of demyelination are associated with areas of viral RNA/antigen [51]. Clinically, mice develop loss of tail tone and a partial to complete hind-limb paralysis. As a result of the clinical and histologic similarities between MHV-induced demyelination and the human demyelinating disease multiple sclerosis (MS), the MHV system is considered a relevant model for studying the underlying immunopathologic mechanisms contributing to immune-mediated demyelinating diseases [51]. A variety of different mechanisms have been postulated to contribute to MHV-induced demyelination. Several studies suggest that MHV-induced demyelination involves immunopathologic responses against viral antigens expressed in infected tissues [30, 31, 37, 47]. Although virus-specific antibody is considered important in suppressing viral recrudescence [84, 85], it may also have a role in promoting demyelination [48]. MHV infection of immunosuppressed or immunodeficient mice results in high titers of virus within the CNS and death but not robust demyelination [53, 105]. Adoptive transfer of MHV-immune splenocytes results in demyelination to the infected recipients, suggesting a role for immune cells in amplifying demyelination [30, 31]. Additional evidence for T cells in contributing to demyelination is provided by Wu et al. [105] who demonstrated that both $CD4^+$ and $CD8^+$ T cells are important in mediating myelin destruction. In support of this are studies derived from our laboratory demonstrating that adoptive transfer of MHV-specific $CD4^+$ or $CD8^+$ T cells to MHV-infected $RAG1^{-/-}$ mice results in demyelination [30, 31]. However, demyelination was more severe in recipients of $CD4^+$ T cell compared to CD8$^+$ T cell recipients, and this supports a more important role for CD4$^+$ T cells in amplifying demyelination in this model. Indeed, we have demonstrated that MHV-infected CD4$^{-/-}$ mice displayed a significant reduction in the severity of demyelination compared to CD8$^{-/-}$ and immunocompetent wildtype mice, suggesting an important role for CD4$^+$ T cells in amplifying the severity of white matter destruction [53].

While T cells are generally considered important in driving demyelination in mice persistently infected with MHV, the mechanisms by which these cells participate in disease may vary and depend upon various factors including the ability to secrete interferon (IFN)-γ [80, 81]. While conventional CD4 and CD8 αβ T cells are generally viewed as the primary T cell type important in disease, γδ T cells have also been shown to participate in demyelination in MHV-infected athymic mice [16]. In addition, we and others have found that macrophages/microglia are also important in contributing to demyelination [29, 32, 53, 59, 105]. The collective evidence points to a role for inflammatory T cells in contributing to macrophage/microglial infiltration and activation which ultimately results in myelin destruction. Current evidence suggests that demyelination in MHV-infected mice is not the result of epitope spreading and induction of an immune response against neuroantigens as has recently been reported to occur during Theiler's virus-induced demyelination [69]. However, adoptive transfer of T cells from MHV-infected rats to naïve recipient's results in demyelination [100]. Whether a similar response occurs in MHV-infected mice and what the contributions are to demyelination is not clear at this time.

1.4
Chemokines and Chemokine Receptors

Chemokines represent a family of low molecular weight (7–17 kDa) proinflammatory cytokines that are divided into four subfamilies based on structural and functional criteria [14, 60, 94]. The two major subfamilies are the CXC and CC chemokines. The CXC subfamily is structurally characterized by two conserved cysteine residues that are separated by an amino acid, while the CC subfamily is structurally characterized by conserved cysteine residues adjacent to one another. Lymphotactin, the sole member of the C family, is chemotactic for T cells [44]. The CX$_3$C chemokine, fractalkine, is unique in that it is expressed on the surface of cells as well as being secreted into the surrounding environment [5].

Chemokines have been shown to selectively attract distinct leukocyte populations during periods of inflammation in various disease models. The CXC chemokines function primarily in attracting neutrophils, yet have a limited effect on T lymphocytes and monocytes [14, 60, 94]. However, there are exceptions to this rule in that CXC chemokines that lack the glutamic acid-leucine-arginine (ELR) motif on the amino terminus are chemotactic for T cells. For example, the non-ELR chemokine CXCL10 is a potent chemoattractant for activated T cells and NK cells and functions by binding to CXCR3 expressed on the surface of these cells [40, 83, 102, 106]. However, CXCL10 does not exert a chemotactic effect on neutrophils [19]. The CC chemokines are thought to attract T cells, monocytes, and macrophages, but not neutrophils [14, 60, 94]. The CC chemokine ligand 5 (CCL5) is able to attract both T cells and macrophages by binding to one of several CC chemokine receptors including CCR1 and CCR5 [14, 60, 94]. Furthermore, there is increasing evidence that chemokines, such as CCL3, influence other immune system activities including T_H1/T_H2 development and T cell proliferation [46, 95]. Chemokines function by binding to seven-transmembrane-spanning G protein-coupled receptors. The chemokine receptors are divided into those that preferentially bind CXC and CC chemokines. In addition, CC and CXC chemokine receptors are capable of binding more than one CC or CXC chemokine, respectively. A variety of cell types including lymphocytes and macrophages, as well as resident cells of the CNS such as neurons, astrocytes, and microglia, express chemokine receptors [60, 94].

2
Orchestrated Expression of Chemokines and Chemokine Receptors Within the CNS Following Infection with MHV

Instillation of MHV into the CNS of susceptible mice results in a well-orchestrated expression of chemokine genes, and the expression pattern correlates with the level of inflammation and disease [52]. Early (~1–3 days) following infection, transcripts for CXCL10 and CCL3 are detected within the CNS, suggesting an important role in initiation of immune responses (see following section; Table 1). By day 6 post-infection (p.i.), virus has spread throughout the brain parenchyma, and a robust inflammatory response, characterized primarily by $CD4^+$ and $CD8^+$ T cells and macrophages, is established within the brain. Chemokines expressed at this time include CXCL9, CXCL10, CCL2, CCL3, CCL4, CCL5, and CCL7 (MIP-2) (Table 1). Analysis of chemokine receptor expression by both RNAse protection assay (RPA), immunostaining, and flow cytometry reveals that CCR1, CCR2, CCR5, and CXCR3 are the prominent receptors expressed within the CNS at various stages of disease (Table 2).

Chemokine transcripts are detected almost exclusively in areas in which virus is present, indicating a localized response to infection and subsequent

Table 1 Chemokine gene expression following MHV infection of the CNS

Days post infection	Chemokine	Function (cells attracted)	Reference(s)
1–3	CXCL10	NK cells	97
	CCL3	Dendritic cells	96
7 and 12	CCL2	Macrophage	39, 52
	CCL3	Dendritic cells, T cells	95, 96
	CCL4		52
	CCL5	T cells, macrophage	52, 53
	CXCL9	T cells	58
	CXCL10	T cells	18, 57
≥21	CXCL10	$CD4^+$ T cells	59
	CCL5	T cells, macrophages	32

Table 2 Chemokine receptors expressed within the CNS of MHV-infected mice

Days post infection	Receptor	Chemokine receptor expression	Reference(s)
1–3	CCR2	T cells, macrophages	13, 39
7 and 12	CCR2	T cells, macrophages	13, 39
	CCR5	T cells, macrophages	29, 30
	CXCR3	T cells	57
>21	CXCR3	T cells	59
	CCR5	T cells, macrophage	29

spread of the virus throughout the parenchyma. In situ hybridization indicates that astrocytes are the primary cellular source for many chemokines during the acute stage of disease [52]. Infection of primary cultures of mouse astrocytes with MHV and evaluating chemokine gene expression by RPA provide additional support for astrocytes as an important cellular source of chemokines in this model [52]. Moreover, viral replication appears to be a necessary prerequisite for inducing chemokine expression, as infection of astrocytes with inactivated virus results in a muted chemokine expression profile. Additional analysis revealed that both infected and noninfected astrocytes are capable of secreting chemokines following instillation of virus into the brain, indicating that viral infection is not required for chemokine gene synthesis by target cells. These data indicate that a factor or factors (possibly type I interferons) derived from infected cells are capable of functioning in both an autocrine and paracrine manner and regulate chemokine gene expression in response to viral infection. Other cell types that may also secrete chemokines following MHV infection include resident microglia/inflammatory macrophages as well as neurons [52, 75].

By day 12 p.i., MHV-infected mice that have survived the acute stage of disease develop an immune-mediated demyelinating disease. Mice have cleared infectious virus (as determined by plaque assay) by 12 days, yet viral RNA and protein can be detected within white matter tracts for months after infection. As the level of CNS infiltration subsides following reduction of viral burden there is a corollary reduction in the expression of chemokine transcripts. Analysis of chemokine message expression within the brains and spinal cords of MHV-infected mice during the demyelinating phase of disease (days 12 and onward) indicates that CXCL10 and CCL5 are the two prominent chemokines expressed [52]. In situ hybridization for chemokine transcripts indicated expression was limited primarily to areas of viral persistence within white matter tracts undergoing active demyelination [52]. Similar to what was found during acute disease, astrocytes were determined to be the cellular source of CXCL10 at this stage of disease whereas inflammatory cells, presumably $CD4^+$ T lymphocytes, expressed CCL5. More recent data now indicate that MHV-infected astrocytes treated with IFN-γ can also express CCL5 mRNA transcripts and protein (T.E. Lane, unpublished observations). Chemokine receptors expressed during chronic demyelination include CXCR3 and CCR5, which are capable of binding CXCL10 and CCL5, respectively. Indeed, we have recently determined that the majority (~90%) of infiltrating virus-specific $CD4^+$ and $CD8^+$ T cells express CXCR3 (T.E. Lane, unpublished observations).

3
Chemokines, Innate Immune Response, and MHV-Infection of the CNS

The presence of dendritic cells (DCs) within the CNS has been debated for quite some time. However, a series of recent studies clearly indicates that during induction of an autoimmune demyelinating disease, there exists the presence of cell types within the brain that clearly have characteristics of DCs [34, 65]. In addition, emerging evidence points to a previously unappreciated role for chemokines in activating and inducing the migration of differing populations of DCs in response to microbial infection of the CNS [22, 23]. These cells may be important in initiation and/or maintenance of disease by participating in the activation of T cells. Given the potential importance of this population of cells with regards to linking innate and adaptive immune responses following viral infection of the CNS, we investigated whether DC-like cells were present within the CNS in response to MHV infection. In brief, our findings clearly indicate that a DC-like population of cells is detectable within the CNS as early as day 2 p.i. with MHV [96]. The activation/maturation of these cells as well as the ability to accumulate within the draining cervical lymph node (CLN) appeared to be dictated by localized expression of CCL3 [96]. Moreover, the ability of cultured DCs to secrete cytokines associated with the development of a T_H1 response such as interleukin (IL)-12 was profoundly altered in the absence of CCL3 [96]. The importance of CCL3 signaling and the evolution of an effective T cell response was further confirmed by the demonstration that in the absence of CCL3 signaling, robust anti-viral effector responses, e.g., cytokine production and CTL activity, were dramatically compromised following MHV infection of CCL3$^{-/-}$ mice [95, 96]. Collectively, these studies highlight a previously unappreciated role for the importance of chemokine signaling and DC maturation/activation following MHV infection of the CNS. Moreover, these studies demonstrate that generation of effective T cell responses relies upon CCL3 signaling to successfully combat MHV infection.

4
Chemokines and Chemokine Receptors and Their Role in Acute Viral-Induced Encephalomyelitis

4.1
CCL3

CCL3 is a chemoattractant for both T cells and macrophages and has been implicated in host defense following infection with a wide variety of microbial pathogens. Mice deficient in CCL3 production exhibit increased susceptibility to disease following infection with paramyxovirus [17], influenza virus [15], and coxsackievirus, as well as other microbial pathogens [67, 72]. In all cases, alterations in an effective host response correlated with a paucity in leukocyte accumulation at sites of infection. Although originally thought to participate in defense by attracting effector cells to infected tissue, recent reports also suggest that CCL3 expression is important in coordinating a T_H1 response [46]. Numerous studies now indicate that DCs are capable of expressing various chemokines including CCL3 [21, 66, 77, 78]. Moreover, DC precursors express the CCL3 receptors CCR1 and CCR5 and are capable of responding to CCL3 in vivo and in vitro resulting in both mobilization and maturation [24, 108]. Indeed, Flesch and colleagues have demonstrated an important role for CCL3 in DC-dependent priming of CTL to viral antigens [24].

Using CCL3$^{-/-}$ mice, we have demonstrated a role for CCL3 in regulating trafficking as well as antiviral effector functions following MHV infection of the CNS [95]. Specifically, our experiments revealed an important role for CCL3 signaling in tailoring T cell responses that allowed for egress out of draining cervical lymph nodes and trafficking into the CNS. Although generation of antigen-specific CD8$^+$ T cells was not impaired following MHV infection of CCL3$^{-/-}$ mice, a significant percentage of CD8$^+$ T cells retained expression of lymph-node homing receptors CD62L (L-selectin) and the CC chemokine receptor 7 (CCR7) and did not display a dramatic increase in mRNA transcripts for either CXCR3 or CCR5, two receptors which are important in allowing MHV-specific T cells access to the CNS [95]. Moreover, adoptive transfer of CCL3$^{-/-}$ CD8$^+$ T cells into MHV-infected RAG1$^{-/-}$ mice (which express CCL3 following MHV infection) resulted in homing back to secondary lymphoid organs, suggesting that lack of CCL3 imprinted on these cells carries an inability to remodulate surface tissue homing receptors. Analysis of antiviral effector functions also revealed that CCL3$^{-/-}$ CD8$^+$ T cells displayed overall muted cytolytic activity as well as expression of IFN-γ when compared to CCL3$^{+/+}$ CD8$^+$ T cells [95]. Collectively, these studies highlight that, in addition to chemotactic function, chemokines influence specific lymphocyte responses and ultimately effector functions that are required for optimal host defense against microbial pathogens.

4.2
CXCL9 and CXCL10

CXCL9 and CXCL10 attract activated T lymphocytes following binding to CXCR3. Analysis of CXCL9 and CXCL10 mRNA expression within the CNS of MHV-infected mice revealed that CXCL10 was clearly detectable by day 1 p.i. and was prominently expressed at days 7, 12, and 35 p.i. [52]. In contrast, CXCL9 transcripts were only detected at days 7 and 12 p.i. [58]. These data suggested that both CXCL9 and CXCL10 might be important in host defense by attracting antiviral T lymphocytes into the CNS. In support of this is the observation that administration of neutralizing antibodies specific for either CXCL9 or CXCL10 to MHV-infected mice during the acute stage of disease results in a dramatic increase in mortality [57, 58]. Additionally, this treatment also resulted in a significant decrease in numbers of CD4$^+$ and CD8$^+$ T lymphocyte infiltrating into the CNS which correlated with decreased expression of IFN-γ and increased levels of virus [57, 58]. MHV infection of CXCL10$^{-/-}$ mice supported and extended our previous work on antibody-mediated neutralization of CXCL10 in that MHV-infected CXCL10$^{-/-}$ mice display reduced T cell infiltration into the CNS accompanied by reduced IFN-γ secretion and increased viral burden [18]. Therefore, the collective evidence points to pivotal roles for both CXCL9 and CXCL10 as important sentinel molecules in promoting a protective response following MHV infection of the CNS by attracting T cells into the CNS that participate in elimination of virus.

4.3
CCL5

CCL5 is a T cell and macrophage chemoattractant that has been shown to influence leukocyte migration during periods of inflammation. Upon MHV infection of the CNS of mice, CCL5 transcripts and protein are readily detected within the brain [52]. Initial studies in which $CD4^{-/-}$ or $CD8^{-/-}$ mice were infected with MHV indicated an overall reduction in CCL5 mRNA transcripts within the brains of $CD4^{-/-}$ mice, suggesting that $CD4^+$ T cells were either a primary cellular source for CCL5 and/or influenced the expression of CCL5 by resident and inflammatory cells [53]. We now know that both inflammatory $CD4^+$ T cells as well as astrocytes are capable of expressing CCL5 following instillation of MHV into the CNS [32, 53]. Furthermore, treatment with neutralizing anti-CCL5 antisera results in diminished T cell and macrophage accumulation within the CNS, suggesting that in this model CCL5 is capable of regulating trafficking of these two populations of cells [32].

4.4
CCR5

CCR5 is a member of the CC chemokine receptor family that is expressed on various hematopoietic cells including lymphocytes and macrophages [86]. Chemokines that are capable of binding to CCR5 include CCL3, CCL4, and CCL5 [7, 68, 86]. Recent studies have clearly indicated that CCR5 expression correlates with leukocyte trafficking to sites of inflammation as well as regulating the immune response following microbial infection. For example, mice deficient in CCR5 ($CCR5^{-/-}$) exhibit altered T cell activity and impaired macrophage function [88, 109]. Furthermore, macrophage trafficking in response to antigen is impaired in $CCR5^{-/-}$ mice, indicating that CCR5 is required for migration of this population of cells [45]. Given that both T cells and macrophages express CCR5 following MHV infection of the CNS and these cells clearly influence outcome in response to infection, we have defined the contributions of CCR5 to both host defense and disease in response to MHV infection. Using an adoptive transfer model in which virus-expanded T cells are transferred into MHV-infected $RAG1^{-/-}$ mice, we have been able to examine how CCR5 expression influences trafficking of T cells into the CNS. Transfer of $CCR5^{+/+}$-derived $CD4^+$ T cells to MHV-infected $RAG1^{-/-}$ mice resulted in $CD4^+$ T cell entry into the CNS and a reduction in viral titers within the brain [30]. These mice also displayed robust demyelination correlating with macrophage accumulation within the CNS. Conversely, $CD4^+$ T cells from $CCR5^{-/-}$ mice displayed an impaired ability to traffic into the CNS of MHV-infected $RAG1^{-/-}$ recipients, which correlated with increased viral titers, diminished macrophage accumulation, and limited demyelination. Analysis of chemokine receptor mRNA expression by M133–147-expanded $CCR5^{-/-}$-derived $CD4^+$ T cells revealed reduced expression of CCR1, CCR2, and CXCR3, indicating that CCR5 signaling is important in increased expression of these receptors which aid in trafficking of $CD4^+$ T cells into the CNS. Collectively these results demonstrate that CCR5 signaling is important to migration of $CD4^+$ T cells to the CNS following MHV infection.

With regards to the role of CCR5 in $CD8^+$ T cell trafficking, comparable numbers of virus-specific $CD8^+$ T cells derived from immunized $CCR5^{+/+}$ or $CCR5^{-/-}$ mice were present within the CNS of MHV-infected $RAG1^{-/-}$ mice following adoptive transfer, indicating that CCR5 is not required for trafficking of these cells into the CNS [30]. $RAG1^{-/-}$ recipients of $CCR5^{-/-}$-derived $CD8^+$ T cells exhibited a modest yet significant ($p \leq 0.05$) reduction in viral burden within the brain that correlated with increased cytolytic activity and IFN-γ expression. Histologic analysis of $RAG1^{-/-}$ recipients of either $CCR5^{+/+}$ or $CCR5^{-/-}$-derived $CD8^+$ T cells revealed only focal areas of demyelination with no significant differences in white matter destruction. These data indicate that CCR5 signaling on virus-specific $CD8^+$ T cells modulates antiviral activities but is not essential for entry into the CNS.

Finally, MHV infection of $CCR5^{-/-}$ mice resulted in a dramatic reduction in macrophage (defined as $CD45^{high}F4/80^+$ dual-positive cells) accumulation within the brains, and this correlated with a significant reduction in the severity of demyelination compared to $CCR5^{+/+}$ mice. Collectively, these data suggest that ligand binding, e.g., CCL5 and/or CCL3, and signaling via CCR5 results in macrophage migration and infiltration into the CNS. However, we have previously demonstrated that CCL3 is expressed only at low levels during acute disease and is not detectable during chronic demyelination, whereas robust expression of CCL5 is detected during both phases of disease, and this suggests that CCL5 is the primary CCR5 signaling chemokine in this model. This is supported by earlier studies that showed an important role for CCL5 in attracting macrophages into the CNS following MHV infection [53]. Therefore, the data presented in this study suggest that one mechanism by which CCL5 contributes to demyelination is via attracting macrophages into the CNS through CCR5-mediated signaling pathways. Additional evidence supporting this is provided by the observation that even in the presence of increased CCL5 expression at day 12 p.i., demyelination is reduced in $CCR5^{-/-}$ mice.

4.5
CCL2 and CCR2

CCL2 is capable of regulating the pathobiology of various inflammatory diseases including MS and atherosclerosis [1, 8, 28, 33, 35, 61]. In addition to its potent chemoattractant effect on monocytes and macrophages, CCL2 also influences T_H2 polarization in response to certain antigenic challenge [36, 41, 46, 99]. The influence of CCL2 on T cell polarization may be due to the fact that CCL2 is constitutively expressed within secondary lymphoid tissue and would be capable of affecting cellular responses following exposure to antigen [36]. Thus, available evidence indicates that expression of CCL2 is capable of influencing both innate as well as adaptive immune responses by regulating monocyte and T cell responses, respectively.

Analysis of chemokine receptor expression following MHV infection reveals that CCR2 is expressed by endogenous cells of the CNS as well as by inflammatory T cells and macrophages, indicating a role for these receptors in regulating both the immune response and disease development [13, 31]. Indeed, MHV-infection of $CCR2^{-/-}$ mice resulted in a dramatic increase in mortality and enhanced viral recovery from the brain that correlated with reduced T cell and macrophage entry into the CNS compared to viral infection of $CCR2^{+/+}$ mice [13].

MHV infection of $CCL2^{-/-}$ mice does not result in a similar disease phenotype as observed in $CCR2^{-/-}$ mice. This was somewhat surprising as CCR2 is currently the only known functional receptor for CCL2. Specifically, $CCL2^{-/-}$ mice were able to clear virus from the brain in a similar time frame as wildtype mice, and this correlated with the ability to generate antigen-specific T cells [39]. The deficiency in $CCR2^{-/-}$ mice to clear virus from the brain is not the result of an inherent inability to generate an effective adaptive immune response to virus, as $CCR2^{-/-}$ mice had a similar frequency of antigen-presenting cells (APC) and virus-specific T cells present within draining CLN compared to either $CCL2^{-/-}$ or wildtype mice. Our findings from MHV infection of $CCL2^{-/-}$ mice indicated that while CCL2 does influence leukocyte migration into the CNS in response to viral infection, CCR2 is clearly more influential in directing T cell trafficking into the CNS. In support of the role for CCL2 in promoting leukocyte migration into the CNS of MHV-infected mice are recent studies by Perlman and colleagues demonstrating that localized CCL2 expression within the CNS promotes macrophage infiltration [47]. These data highlight the possibility that ligand(s) other than CCL2 are important in signaling through the CCR2 receptor. Alternatively, it is possible that CCR2 signaling by either endothelial cells and/or astrocytes regulates the permeability of the BBB, as recently suggested by Stamatovic and colleagues [91].

5
Chemokines and Chronic Viral-Induced Demyelination

Expression of chemokines has been associated with demyelinating plaque lesions present in MS patients [3, 4, 26, 27]. Elevated levels of chemokines, notably CXCL10, were found in the cerebral spinal fluid (CSF) of MS patients during periods of clinical attack [25, 89]. Indeed, the concentration of CXCL10 within the CSF of MS patients correlated with numbers of inflammatory cells and the severity of clinical disease [2, 89, 90]. Moreover, when CXCL10 levels decreased, there was a corresponding decrease in inflammation and disease severity [89]. Astrocyte expression of CXCL10 has been reported in active plaque lesions present in MS patients, and the majority of T cells infiltrating into the CNS of MS patients express the CXCL10 receptor, CXCR3. Collectively, these studies highlight a potentially important role for CXCL10 in the pathogenesis of demyelinating diseases such as MS by attracting CXCR3-expressing T cells into the CNS and support targeting chemokines and their receptors for therapeutic intervention in the treatment of MS [10, 54, 70, 90].

Studies from animal models of MS support this notion by demonstrating that blocking of CXCL10 often results in diminished disease severity accompanied by a marked reduction in neuroinflammation. For example, several recent reports indicate that treatment with anti-CXCL10 neutralizing antibodies resulted in delayed disease onset and diminished neuroinflammation in mice with the autoimmune demyelinating disease experimental autoimmune encephalomyelitis (EAE) [20]. These studies support the idea that localized expression of CXCL10 within the CNS amplifies disease severity by attracting CXCR3-expressing T cells into the CNS. Once present, these cells enhance neuroinflammation by secreting additional chemokines as well as cytokines that can activate resident glia cells. Importantly, these studies also implicate CXCL10 as a potential therapeutic target and suggest that alternative CXCR3 ligands, e.g., CXCL9 and CXCL11, do not exert a prominent effect on T cell infiltration into the CNS. However, the role of CXCL10 in contributing to neurologic disease in EAE has been questioned by results indicating that CXCL10 may actually exert a protective effect in mice with EAE [49, 71]. Antibody-mediated neutralization following induction of EAE in rats resulted in increased disease severity, and this was associated with smaller draining lymph nodes and increased numbers of $CD4^+$ T cells infiltrating into the CNS [71]. In addition, $CXCL10^{-/-}$ mice exhibited increased clinical disease severity following immunization with myelin peptides, and this correlated with diminished lymph node sizes although T cell infiltration into the CNS was not dramatically altered when compared to wildtype mice [49]. In these particular EAE models in which mice are immunized peripherally with antigen, CXCL10 expression within secondary lymphoid tissue is considered important in dictating disease outcome by serving to retain lymphocytes and tailoring T cell responses. Moreover, these findings highlight the different roles of CXCL10 in regulating cellular immune responses in different models of neuroinflammation and emphasize the need for a better understanding of how signaling by this chemokine regulates inflammation and disease.

As indicated, we have determined that MHV infection of the CNS results in an orchestrated expression of chemokine and chemokine receptor genes that are regulated, in large part, by the viral burden. Similar to MS patients, CXCL10 is expressed primarily by astrocytes in areas undergoing demyelination, suggesting an important role in the pathogenesis of demyelination by attracting CXCR3-expressing T cells into the CNS [52, 59]. Indeed, our laboratory was the first to demonstrate that treatment of mice with established demyelination and paralysis with anti-CXCL10 neutralizing antibody resulted in a significant reduction in $CD4^+$—but not $CD8^+$—T cells present within the CNS, and this correlated with improved motor skills and a reduction in the severity of demyelination [59]. Moreover, the dramatic regain of movement in anti-CXCL10-treated mice corresponded with more than 80% of previously demyelinated axons undergoing remyelination, indicating that removal of CXCL10 promoted an environment capable of remyelination. In addition to reduced numbers of $CD4^+$ T cells within the CNS, there was a paucity of macrophage infiltration into the CNS of anti-CXCL10-treated mice that correlated with a dramatic reduction in the levels of the macrophage-chemoattractant CCL5. These data were consistent with previous studies indicating that $CD4^+$ T cells were the major source for CCL5 in MHV-infected mice undergoing demyelination [53, 59]. The influence of CXCL10 in contributing to T cell responses was also examined. T cells isolated from secondary lymphoid tissue of mice treated with anti-CXCL10 displayed muted expression of IFN-γ in response to viral antigen when compared to T cells isolated from control mice, suggesting that CXCL10 also serves to influence T cell effector functions during chronic disease (T.E. Lane, unpublished observations).

We have previously determined that CCL5 mRNA transcripts and protein are present within the CNS of MHV-infected mice during chronic demyelination, indicating a potentially important role for this chemokine in promoting inflammation [52, 53]. In order to assess the functional role of CCL5 in participating in viral-induced immune-mediated demyelination, MHV-infected mice were treated via intraperitoneal (i.p.) injection with anti-CCL5 monoclonal antibody (mAb) following onset of clinical disease and demyelination. Such treatment resulted in a significant ($p \leq 0.05$) reduction in the severity of clinical disease compared to mice treated with an isotype (IgG_1)-matched antibody [32]. Upon removal of anti-CCL5 treatment, clinical disease returned to mice such that there was no difference between the two experimental groups of mice. Immunophenotyping the cellular infiltrate of mice treated with anti-CCL5 revealed reduced T cell and macrophage infiltration into the CNS that is consistent with our earlier studies that CCL5 attracts these cells into the CNS of mice with chronic demyelination. Further, analysis of the severity of demyelination in experimental groups of mice indicated that anti-CCL5 treatment resulted in a significant ($p<0.05$) reduction in the severity of demyelination compared to control-treated mice.

A picture is slowly evolving from our experiments designed to test the functional contributions of CXCL10 and CCL5 to chronic demyelination within MHV-infected mice. Antibody targeting of the T cell chemoattractant CXCL10 in MHV-infected mice selectively affects $CD4^+$ T cell accumulation within the CNS accompanied by improved motor skills and a reduction in the severity of demyelination [59]. In contrast, CCL5 is capable of attracting both $CD4^+$ and $CD8^+$ T cells into the CNS. It is also important to emphasize that our data on CCL5 and CXCL10 inhibition with regards to T cell and macrophage trafficking are corollary and it is possible that alternative scenarios exist. For example, studies by Bergmann and colleagues suggest that during persistent MHV infection there is limited to no trafficking of T cells from the periphery into the CNS. Rather, upon entry during acute encephalomyelitis a certain percentage of $CD4^+$ and $CD8^+$ T cells is retained and participate in disease [62, 93]. In this instance, CXCL10 expression would not be functioning as a T cell chemoattractant but rather to influence specific biologic functions of T cells as well as potentiating the retention of T cells within the CNS. In support of this, it is possible that CXCL10 serves to enhance $CD4^+$ T cell proliferation, as several recent studies indicate that CXCL10 is important in contributing to T cell proliferation [18, 71, 101].

It is unlikely that CXCL10 contributes to T cell survival, as $CXCL10^{-/-}$ mice do not display any abnormalities with regards to T cell half-life nor do we see any increase in numbers of apoptotic T cells following anti-CXCL10 treatment. In addition, Narumi et al. [71] speculate that CXCL10 actually serves to retain $CXCR3^+$ T cells within tissues and this influences disease severity. Therefore, the selective reduction in $CD4^+$ T cells within the CNS of MHV-infected mice may not be the result of impaired trafficking. Rather, either $CD4^+$ T cells are not undergoing a steady-state turnover or are actually migrating out of the CNS in the absence of signals specifying their retention.

In addition, recent studies indicate an important role for CXCL10 in imparting effector functions to T cells. For example, Salomon and colleagues demonstrated that anti-CXCL10 treatment improved joint swelling in a rodent model of arthritis and this correlated in part with an altered T_H1/T_H2 balance, suggesting that CXCL10 expression promotes and maintains a T_H1 state in T cells in this model [87].

Similarly, we have shown that MHV-infection of CXCL10$^{-/-}$ mice results in diminished IFN-γ expression by virus-specific T cells, supporting the idea that CXCL10 expression serves to maintain a T_H1-like state in T cells [18] (T.E. Lane, unpublished observations). CCL5 signaling also modulates cytokine production by T cells following antigenic challenge. In support of this is our demonstration that inhibition of CCL5 signaling results in enhanced IFN-γ expression by virus-specific T cells, supporting the idea that CCL5 expression serves to regulate a T_H1-like state in T cells [32]. Moreover, ablation of CCL5 signaling also modifies the cytolytic activity of MHV-specific CD8$^+$ T cells [30].

6
Perspectives

This chapter highlights mechanisms by which chemokines participate in both host defense and disease progression in response to MHV infection of the CNS. An overview of the potential functional role for select chemokines in linking innate and adaptive immune responses in response to viral infection of the CNS is provided in Fig. 1. In brief, following MHV infection there is robust expression of chemokines by infected astrocytes including CCL3 that contribute to the maturation/activation of local DCs, which ultimately enables migration to draining cervical lymph nodes. Activated DCs present antigen to T cells as well as secrete chemokines such as CCL3 and CXCL10 that enhance polarization to a T_H1 response. In turn, MHV-specific T cells express chemokine receptors including CXCR3 and CCR5 that enable them to traffic into the CNS as a result of localized expression of ligands CXCL9 and CXCL10 (ligands for CXCR3) as well as CCL5 (ligand for CCR5). In addition, our contention is that expression of CCR2 by endothelial cells of the BBB is also important in increasing the permeability of this structure.

With regards to chronic disease, MHV persistence within the CNS results in chronic expression of CXCL10 and CCL5 which together contribute to the maintenance of a chronic inflammatory disease by attracting both T cells and macrophages (Fig. 2). Local secretion of CXCL10 and CCL5 may also contribute to demyelination by enhancing specific T cell effector functions including (1) secretion of IFN-γ that activates local inflammatory macrophage and resident microglia, as well as directly damaging oligodendrocytes and (2) increasing CTL activity by CD8$^+$ T cells.

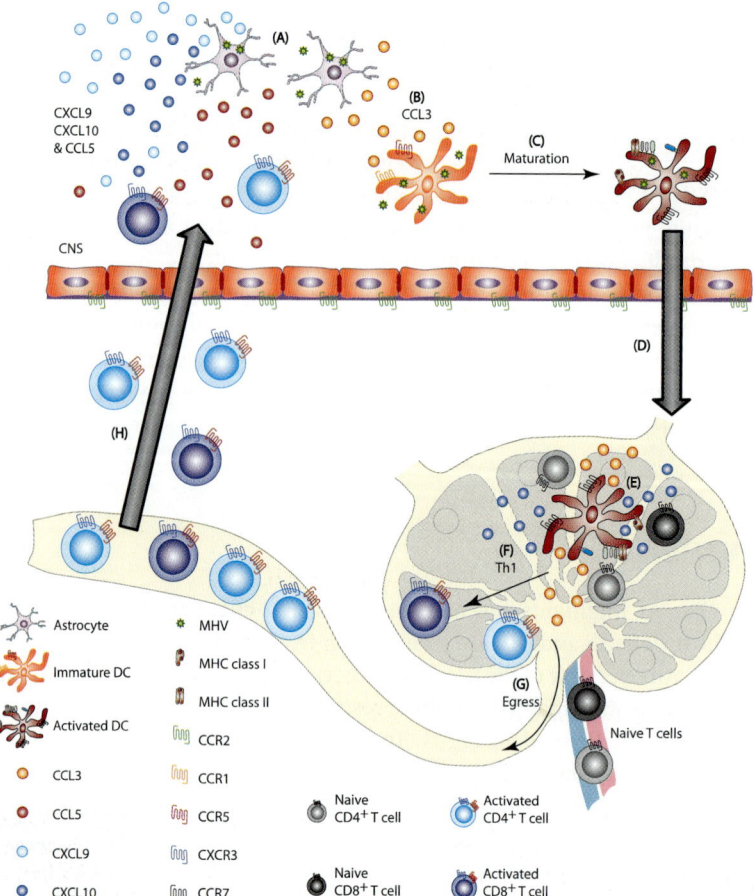

Fig. 1A–H Chemokines and innate/adaptive immune response following MHV infection of the CNS. Instillation of MHV into the CNS of susceptible mice results in infection of astrocytes that are an important source of chemokines including CXCL10, CCL5, and CCL3 (**A**). In addition, immature DC-like cells may also be susceptible to infection and secrete CCL3 (**B**) that functions in a paracrine and autocrine manner to bind to CCR1 expressed on immature DC-like cells. As a result of CCL3 signaling and MHV infection, the DC-like cells undergo maturation and activation (**C**) resulting in a remodulation of the plasma membrane characterized by decreased expression of CCR1 accompanied by increased expression of CCR7 as well as major histocompatibility complex (MHC) class I and II. CCR7-expressing, activated DCs home to the draining cervical lymph node (**D**). Upon entry, activated DCs express a variety of soluble factors including CCL3 and CXCL10 (**E**) that activate and enhance polarization of virus-specific T cells to a T_H1 phenotype (**F**). Activated T cells exit the lymph node via the efferent lymph (**G**), enter the blood stream, and migrate to the CNS via expression of the chemokine receptors CXCR3 and CCR5 (**H**)

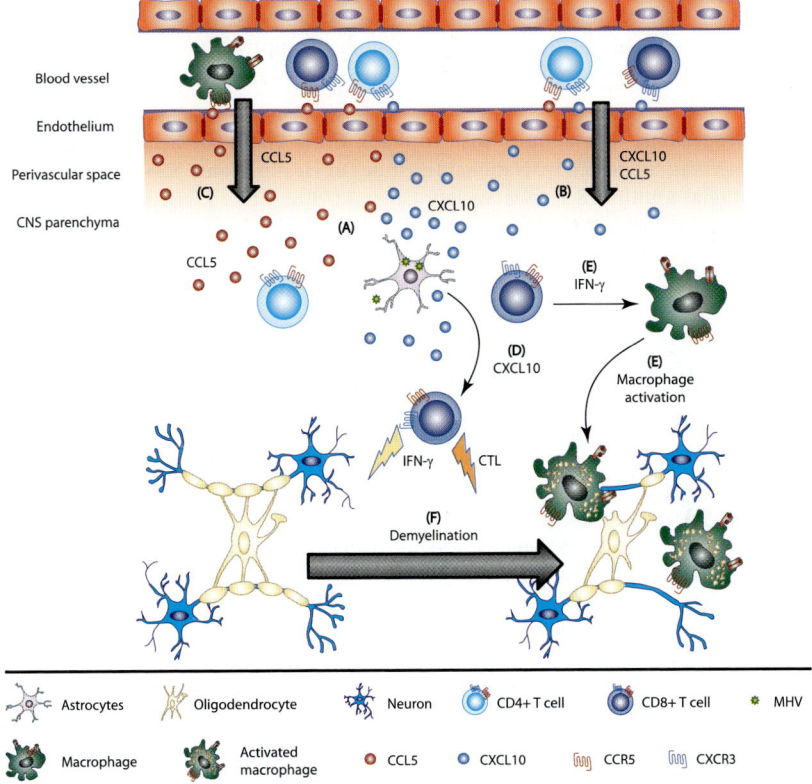

Fig. 2A–F Chemokines and MHV-induced demyelination. Persistent MHV infection within astrocytes leads to chronic CXCL10 and CCL5 expression (**A**) that serves to recruit CXCR3$^+$ and CCR5$^+$ T cells into the CNS (**B**). In addition, activated CD4$^+$ T cells secrete CCL5 that enhances macrophage migration into the CNS (**C**). We believe that CXCL10 may also influence T cell effector functions within the CNS, including CTL activity (**D**) and IFN-γ secretion (**E**), leading to macrophage activation. Both IFN-γ production and CTL activity may enhance tissue destruction as well as macrophage activation that amplifies myelin destruction (**F**)

Clearly, these observations indicate that chemokine signaling is an integral component involved in eliciting protective immunity in response to viral infection of the CNS. Conversely, our studies also indicate that chronic localized secretion of select chemokines ultimately amplifies disease severity through maintaining inflammation within the CNS. Importantly, studies derived from the MHV system demonstrate that antibody targeting of select chemokines offers a powerful approach towards delineating the functional contributions of these molecules in a model of immune-mediated demyelination. Further, these studies highlight the relevancy of such an approach in treating human neuroinflammatory and demyelinating diseases such as MS.

Acknowledgements The authors wish to thank Craig Walsh for helpful discussion. This work was supported by National Institutes of Health grants NS41249, NS18146, and National Multiple Sclerosis Society Grant 3278 to T.E.L. J.L.H. is supported by postdoctoral fellowship 1652 from the National Multiple Sclerosis Society.

References

1. Baggiolini M (2001) Chemokines in pathology and medicine. J Intern Med 250:91–104
2. Balashov KE, Rottman JB, Weiner HL, Hancock WW (1999) CCR5(+) and CXCR3(+) T cells are increased in multiple sclerosis and their ligands MIP-1alpha and IP-10 are expressed in demyelinating brain lesions. Proc Natl Acad Sci U S A 96:6873–6878
3. Banisor I, Leist TP, Kalman B (2005) Involvement of beta-chemokines in the development of inflammatory demyelination. J Neuroinflammation 2:7
4. Bartosik-Psujek H, Stelmasiak Z (2005) The levels of chemokines CXCL8, CCL2 and CCL5 in multiple sclerosis patients are linked to the activity of the disease. Eur J Neurol 12:49–54
5. Bazan JF, Bacon KB, Hardiman G, Wang W, Soo K, Rossi D, Greaves DR, Zlotnik A, Schall TJ (1997) A new class of membrane-bound chemokine with a CX3C motif. Nature 385:640–644
6. Biron CA, Nguyen KB, Pien GC, Cousens LP, Salazar-Mather TP (1999) Natural killer cells in antiviral defense: function and regulation by innate cytokines. Annu Rev Immunol 17:189–220
7. Boring L, Gosling J, Monteclaro FS, Lusis AJ, Tsou CL, Charo IF (1996) Molecular cloning and functional expression of murine JE (monocyte chemoattractant protein 1) and murine macrophage inflammatory protein 1alpha receptors: evidence for two closely linked C-C chemokine receptors on chromosome 9. J Biol Chem 271:7551–7558
8. Boring L, Gosling J, Cleary M, Charo IF (1998) Decreased lesion formation in $^{-/-}$CCR2$-/-$ mice reveals a role for chemokines in the initiation of atherosclerosis. Nature 394:894–897
9. Buchmeier MJ, Lewicki HA, Talbot PJ, Knobler RL (1984) Murine hepatitis virus-4 (strain JHM)-induced neurologic disease is modulated in vivo by monoclonal antibody. Virology 132:261–270
10. Cartier L, Hartley O, Dubois-Dauphin M, Krause KH (2005) Chemokine receptors in the central nervous system: role in brain inflammation and neurodegenerative diseases. Brain Res Brain Res Rev 48:16–42
11. Castro RF, Perlman S (1995) CD8+ T-cell epitopes within the surface glycoprotein of a neurotropic coronavirus and correlation with pathogenicity. J Virol 69:8127–8131

12. Cheever FS, Daniels JB, Pappenheimer AM, Bailey OT (1949) A murine virus (JHM) causing disseminated encephalomyelitis with extensive destruction of myelin. J Exp Med 90:181–194
13. Chen BP, Kuziel WA, Lane TE (2001) Lack of CCR2 results in increased mortality and impaired leukocyte activation and trafficking following infection of the central nervous system with a neurotropic coronavirus. J Immunol 167:4585–4592
14. Clark-Lewis I, Kim KS, Rajarathnam K, Gong JH, Dewald B, Moser B, Baggiolini M, Sykes BD (1995) Structure-activity relationships of chemokines. J Leukoc Biol 57:703–711
15. Cook DN, Beck MA, Coffman TM, Kirby SL, Sheridan JF, Pragnell IB, Smithies O (1995) Requirement of MIP-1 alpha for an inflammatory response to viral infection. Science 269:1583–1585
16. Dandekar AA, Perlman S (2002) Virus-induced demyelination in nude mice is mediated by gamma delta T cells. Am J Pathol 161:1255–1263
17. Domachowske JB, Bonville CA, Gao JL, Murphy PM, Easton AJ, Rosenberg HF (2000) The chemokine macrophage-inflammatory protein-1 alpha and its receptor CCR1 control pulmonary inflammation and antiviral host defense in paramyxovirus infection. J Immunol 165:2677–2682
18. Dufour JH, Dziejman M, Liu MT, Leung JH, Lane TE, Luster AD (2002) IFN-gamma-inducible protein 10 (IP-10; CXCL10)-deficient mice reveal a role for IP-10 in effector T cell generation and trafficking. J Immunol 168:3195–3204
19. Farber JM (1997) Mig and IP-10: CXC chemokines that target lymphocytes. J Leukoc Biol 61:246–257
20. Fife BT, Kennedy KJ, Paniagua MC, Lukacs NW, Kunkel SL, Luster AD, Karpus WJ (2001) CXCL10 (IFN-gamma-inducible protein-10) control of encephalitogenic CD4+ T cell accumulation in the central nervous system during experimental autoimmune encephalomyelitis. J Immunol 166:7617–7624
21. Fischer FR, Luo Y, Luo M, Santambrogio L, Dorf ME (2001) RANTES-induced chemokine cascade in dendritic cells. J Immunol 167:1637–1643
22. Fischer HG, Bonifas U, Reichmann G (2000) Phenotype and functions of brain dendritic cells emerging during chronic infection of mice with Toxoplasma gondii. J Immunol 164:4826–4834
23. Fischer HG, Reichmann G (2001) Brain dendritic cells and macrophages/microglia in central nervous system inflammation. J Immunol 166:2717–2726
24. Flesch IE, Stober D, Schirmbeck R, Reimann J (2000) Monocyte inflammatory protein-1 alpha facilitates priming of CD8(+) T cell responses to exogenous viral antigen. Int Immunol 12:1365–1370
25. Franciotta D, Martino G, Zardini E, Furlan R, Bergamaschi R, Andreoni L, Cosi V (2001) Serum and CSF levels of MCP-1 and IP-10 in multiple sclerosis patients with acute and stable disease and undergoing immunomodulatory therapies. J Neuroimmunol 115:192–198
26. Gade-Andavolu R, Comings DE, MacMurray J, Vuthoori RK, Tourtellotte WW, Nagra RM, Cone LA (2004) RANTES: a genetic risk marker for multiple sclerosis. Mult Scler 10:536–539
27. Galimberti D, Bresolin N, Scarpini E (2004) Chemokine network in multiple sclerosis: role in pathogenesis and targeting for future treatments. Expert Rev Neurother 4:439–453

28. Gerard C, Rollins BJ (2001) Chemokines and disease. Nat Immunol 2:108–115
29. Glass WG, Liu MT, Kuziel WA, Lane TE (2001) Reduced macrophage infiltration and demyelination in mice lacking the chemokine receptor CCR5 following infection with a neurotropic coronavirus. Virology 288:8–17
30. Glass WG, Lane TE (2003) Functional analysis of the CC chemokine receptor 5 (CCR5) on virus-specific CD8+ T cells following coronavirus infection of the central nervous system. Virology 312:407–414
31. Glass WG, Lane TE (2003) Functional expression of chemokine receptor CCR5 on CD4(+) T cells during virus-induced central nervous system disease. J Virol 77:191–198
32. Glass WG, Hickey MJ, Hardison JL, Liu MT, Manning JE, Lane TE (2004) Antibody targeting of the CC chemokine ligand 5 results in diminished leukocyte infiltration into the central nervous system and reduced neurologic disease in a viral model of multiple sclerosis. J Immunol 172:4018–4025
33. Gosling J, Slaymaker S, Gu L, Tseng S, Zlot CH, Young SG, Rollins BJ, Charo IF (1999) MCP-1 deficiency reduces susceptibility to atherosclerosis in mice that overexpress human apolipoprotein B. J Clin Invest 103:773–778
34. Greter M, Heppner FL, Lemos MP, Odermatt BM, Goebels N, Laufer T, Noelle RJ, Becher B (2005) Dendritic cells permit immune invasion of the CNS in an animal model of multiple sclerosis. Nat Med 11:328–334
35. Gu L, Tseng SC, Rollins BJ (1999) Monocyte chemoattractant protein-1. Chem Immunol 72:7–29
36. Gu L, Tseng S, Horner RM, Tam C, Loda M, Rollins BJ (2000) Control of TH2 polarization by the chemokine monocyte chemoattractant protein-1. Nature 404:407–411
37. Haring JS, Pewe LL, Perlman S (2001) High-magnitude, virus-specific CD4 T-cell response in the central nervous system of coronavirus-infected mice. J Virol 75:3043–3047
38. Haring JS, Perlman S (2003) Bystander CD4 T cells do not mediate demyelination in mice infected with a neurotropic coronavirus. J Neuroimmunol 137:42–50
39. Held KS, Chen BP, Kuziel WA, Rollins BJ, Lane TE (2004) Differential roles of CCL2 and CCR2 in host defense to coronavirus infection. Virology 329:251–260
40. Hildebrandt GC, Corrion LA, Olkiewicz KM, Lu B, Lowler K, Duffner UA, Moore BB, Kuziel WA, Liu C, Cooke KR (2004) Blockade of CXCR3 receptor:ligand interactions reduces leukocyte recruitment to the lung and the severity of experimental idiopathic pneumonia syndrome. J Immunol 173:2050–2059
41. Hogaboam CM, Lukacs NW, Chensue SW, Strieter RM, Kunkel SL (1998) Monocyte chemoattractant protein-1 synthesis by murine lung fibroblasts modulates CD4+ T cell activation. J Immunol 160:4606–4614
42. Holmes K, Lai M (1996) Coronaviridae: the viruses and their replication. In: Fields BN, Knipe DM, Howley PM (eds) Fields virology. Lippincott-Raven Publishers, New York, pp 1075–1094
43. Holmes KV (2003) SARS-associated coronavirus. N Engl J Med 348:1948–1951
44. Houck JC, Chang CM (1977) The purification and characterization of a lymphokine chemotactic for lymphocytes—lymphotactin. Inflammation 2:105–113

45. Huffnagle GB, McNeil LK, McDonald RA, Murphy JW, Toews GB, Maeda N, Kuziel WA (1999) Cutting edge: role of C-C chemokine receptor 5 in organ-specific and innate immunity to Cryptococcus neoformans. J Immunol 163:4642–4646
46. Karpus WJ, Lukacs NW, Kennedy KJ, Smith WS, Hurst SD, Barrett TA (1997) Differential CC chemokine-induced enhancement of T helper cell cytokine production. J Immunol 158:4129–4136
47. Kim TS, Perlman S (2005) Viral expression of CCL2 is sufficient to induce demyelination in $^{-/-}$RAG1–/– mice infected with a neurotropic coronavirus. J Virol 79:7113–7120
48. Kim TS, Perlman S (2005) Virus-specific antibody, in the absence of T cells, mediates demyelination in mice infected with a neurotropic coronavirus. Am J Pathol 166:801–809
49. Klein RS, Izikson L, Means T, Gibson HD, Lin E, Sobel RA, Weiner HL, Luster AD (2004) IFN-inducible protein 10/CXC chemokine ligand 10-independent induction of experimental autoimmune encephalomyelitis. J Immunol 172:550–559
50. Lai MM, Cavanagh D (1997) The molecular biology of coronaviruses. Adv Virus Res 48:1–100
51. Lane TE, Buchmeier MJ (1997) Murine coronavirus infection: a paradigm for virus-induced demyelinating disease. Trends Microbiol 5:9–14
52. Lane TE, Asensio VC, Yu N, Paoletti AD, Campbell IL, Buchmeier MJ (1998) Dynamic regulation of alpha- and beta-chemokine expression in the central nervous system during mouse hepatitis virus-induced demyelinating disease. J Immunol 160:970–978
53. Lane TE, Liu MT, Chen BP, Asensio VC, Samawi RM, Paoletti AD, Campbell IL, Kunkel SL, Fox HS, Buchmeier MJ (2000) A central role for CD4(+) T cells and RANTES in virus-induced central nervous system inflammation and demyelination. J Virol 74:1415–1424
54. Lazzeri E, Romagnani P (2005) CXCR3-binding chemokines: novel multifunctional therapeutic targets. Curr Drug Targets Immune Endocr Metabol Disord 5:109–118
55. Lin MT, Stohlman SA, Hinton DR (1997) Mouse hepatitis virus is cleared from the central nervous systems of mice lacking perforin-mediated cytolysis. J Virol 71:383–391
56. Lin MT, Hinton DR, Marten NW, Bergmann CC, Stohlman SA (1999) Antibody prevents virus reactivation within the central nervous system. J Immunol 162:7358–7368
57. Liu MT, Chen BP, Oertel P, Buchmeier MJ, Armstrong D, Hamilton TA, Lane TE (2000) The T cell chemoattractant IFN-inducible protein 10 is essential in host defense against viral-induced neurologic disease. J Immunol 165:2327–2330
58. Liu MT, Armstrong D, Hamilton TA, Lane TE (2001) Expression of Mig (monokine induced by interferon-gamma) is important in T lymphocyte recruitment and host defense following viral infection of the central nervous system. J Immunol 166:1790–1795
59. Liu MT, Keirstead HS, Lane TE (2001) Neutralization of the chemokine CXCL10 reduces inflammatory cell invasion and demyelination and improves neurological function in a viral model of multiple sclerosis. J Immunol 167:4091–4097

60. Luster AD (1998) Chemokines—chemotactic cytokines that mediate inflammation. N Engl J Med 338:436–445
61. Mahad DJ, Ransohoff RM (2003) The role of MCP-1 (CCL2) and CCR2 in multiple sclerosis and experimental autoimmune encephalomyelitis (EAE). Semin Immunol 15:23–32
62. Marten NW, Stohlman SA, Bergmann CC (2000) Role of viral persistence in retaining CD8(+) T cells within the central nervous system. J Virol 74:7903–7910
63. Matsui M, Araya SI, Wang HY, Matsushima K, Saida T (2005) Differences in systemic and central nervous system cellular immunity relevant to relapsing-remitting multiple sclerosis. J Neurol 252:908–915
64. McIntosh K (1996) Diagnostic virology. In: Fields BN, Knipe DM, Howley PM (eds) Fields virology. Lippincott-Raven Publishers, New York, pp 401–430
65. McMahon EJ, Bailey SL, Castenada CV, Waldner H, Miller SD (2005) Epitope spreading initiates in the CNS in two mouse models of multiple sclerosis. Nat Med 11:335–339
66. Megjugorac NJ, Young HA, Amrute SB, Olshalsky SL, Fitzgerald-Bocarsly P (2004) Virally stimulated plasmacytoid dendritic cells produce chemokines and induce migration of T and NK cells. J Leukoc Biol 75:504–514
67. Mehrad B, Moore TA, Standiford TJ (2000) Macrophage inflammatory protein-1 alpha is a critical mediator of host defense against invasive pulmonary aspergillosis in neutropenic hosts. J Immunol 165:962–968
68. Meyer A, Coyle AJ, Proudfoot AE, Wells TN, Power CA (1996) Cloning and characterization of a novel murine macrophage inflammatory protein-1 alpha receptor. J Biol Chem 271:14445–14451
69. Miller SD, Vanderlugt CL, Begolka WS, Pao W, Yauch RL, Neville KL, Katz-Levy Y, Carrizosa A, Kim BS (1997) Persistent infection with Theiler's virus leads to CNS autoimmunity via epitope spreading. Nat Med 3:1133–1136
70. Muller DM, Pender MP, Greer JM (2004) Chemokines and chemokine receptors: potential therapeutic targets in multiple sclerosis. Curr Drug Targets Inflamm Allergy 3:279–290
71. Narumi S, Kaburaki T, Yoneyama H, Iwamura H, Kobayashi Y, Matsushima K (2002) Neutralization of IFN-inducible protein 10/CXCL10 exacerbates experimental autoimmune encephalomyelitis. Eur J Immunol 32:1784–1791
72. Olszewski MA, Huffnagle GB, McDonald RA, Lindell DM, Moore BB, Cook DN, Toews GB (2000) The role of macrophage inflammatory protein-1 alpha/CCL3 in regulation of T cell-mediated immunity to Cryptococcus neoformans infection. J Immunol 165:6429–6436
73. Parra B, Hinton DR, Marten NW, Bergmann CC, Lin MT, Yang CS, Stohlman SA (1999) IFN-gamma is required for viral clearance from central nervous system oligodendroglia. J Immunol 162:1641–1647
74. Parra B, Lin MT, Stohlman SA, Bergmann CC, Atkinson R, Hinton DR (2000) Contributions of Fas-Fas ligand interactions to the pathogenesis of mouse hepatitis virus in the central nervous system. J Virol 74:2447–2450
75. Patterson CE, Daley JK, Echols LA, Lane TE, Rall GF (2003) Measles virus infection induces chemokine synthesis by neurons. J Immunol 171:3102–3109

76. Pearce BD, Hobbs MV, McGraw TS, Buchmeier MJ (1994) Cytokine induction during T-cell-mediated clearance of mouse hepatitis virus from neurons in vivo. J Virol 68:5483–5495
77. Penna G, Vulcano M, Roncari A, Facchetti F, Sozzani S, Adorini L (2002) Cutting edge: differential chemokine production by myeloid and plasmacytoid dendritic cells. J Immunol 169:6673–6676
78. Penna G, Vulcano M, Sozzani S, Adorini L (2002) Differential migration behavior and chemokine production by myeloid and plasmacytoid dendritic cells. Hum Immunol 63:1164–1171
79. Perlman SR, Lane TE, Buchmeier MJ (1999) Coronaviruses: hepatitis, peritonitis and central nervous system disease. In: Cunningham MW, Fujinami RS (eds) Effects of microbes on the immune system, vol. 1. Lippincott Williams and Wilkins, Philadelphia, pp 331–348
80. Pewe L, Haring J, Perlman S (2002) CD4 T-cell-mediated demyelination is increased in the absence of gamma interferon in mice infected with mouse hepatitis virus. J Virol 76:7329–7333
81. Pewe L, Perlman S (2002) Cutting edge: CD8 T cell-mediated demyelination is IFN-gamma dependent in mice infected with a neurotropic coronavirus. J Immunol 168:1547–1551
82. Phillips JJ, Chua M, Seo SH, Weiss SR (2001) Multiple regions of the murine coronavirus spike glycoprotein influence neurovirulence. J Neurovirol 7:421–431
83. Qin S, Rottman JB, Myers P, Kassam N, Weinblatt M, Loetscher M, Koch AE, Moser B, Mackay CR (1998) The chemokine receptors CXCR3 and CCR5 mark subsets of T cells associated with certain inflammatory reactions. J Clin Invest 101:746–754
84. Ramakrishna C, Stohlman SA, Atkinson RD, Shlomchik MJ, Bergmann CC (2002) Mechanisms of central nervous system viral persistence: the critical role of antibody and B cells. J Immunol 168:1204–1211
85. Ramakrishna C, Bergmann CC, Atkinson R, Stohlman SA (2003) Control of central nervous system viral persistence by neutralizing antibody. J Virol 77:4670–4678
86. Raport CJ, Gosling J, Schweickart VL, Gray PW, Charo IF (1996) Molecular cloning and functional characterization of a novel human CC chemokine receptor (CCR5) for RANTES, MIP-1beta, and MIP-1alpha. J Biol Chem 271:17161–17166
87. Salomon I, Netzer N, Wildbaum G, Schif-Zuck S, Maor G, Karin N (2002) Targeting the function of IFN-gamma-inducible protein 10 suppresses ongoing adjuvant arthritis. J Immunol 169:2685–2693
88. Sato N, Kuziel WA, Melby PC, Reddick RL, Kostecki V, Zhao W, Maeda N, Ahuja SK, Ahuja SS (1999) Defects in the generation of IFN-gamma are overcome to control infection with Leishmania donovani in CC chemokine receptor (CCR) 5-, macrophage inflammatory protein-1 alpha-, or CCR2-deficient mice. J Immunol 163:5519–5525
89. Sorensen TL, Tani M, Jensen J, Pierce V, Lucchinetti C, Folcik VA, Qin S, Rottman J, Sellebjerg F, Strieter RM, Frederiksen JL, Ransohoff RM (1999) Expression of specific chemokines and chemokine receptors in the central nervous system of multiple sclerosis patients. J Clin Invest 103:807–815

90. Sorensen TL, Trebst C, Kivisakk P, Klaege KL, Majmudar A, Ravid R, Lassmann H, Olsen DB, Strieter RM, Ransohoff RM, Sellebjerg F (2002) Multiple sclerosis: a study of CXCL10 and CXCR3 co-localization in the inflamed central nervous system. J Neuroimmunol 127:59–68
91. Stamatovic SM, Shakui P, Keep RF, Moore BB, Kunkel SL, Van Rooijen N, Andjelkovic AV (2005) Monocyte chemoattractant protein-1 regulation of blood-brain barrier permeability. J Cereb Blood Flow Metab 25:593–606
92. Stohlman SA, Bergmann CC, Lin MT, Cua DJ, Hinton DR (1998) CTL effector function within the central nervous system requires CD4+ T cells. J Immunol 160:2896–2904
93. Stohlman SA, Ramakrishna C, Tschen SI, Hinton DR, Bergmann CC (2002) The art of survival during viral persistence. J Neurovirol 8[Suppl 2]:53–58
94. Taub DD, Oppenheim JJ (1994) Chemokines, inflammation and the immune system. Ther Immunol 1:229–246
95. Trifilo MJ, Bergmann CC, Kuziel WA, Lane TE (2003) CC chemokine ligand 3 (CCL3) regulates CD8(+)-T-cell effector function and migration following viral infection. J Virol 77:4004–4014
96. Trifilo MJ, Lane TE (2004) The CC chemokine ligand 3 regulates CD11c+CD11b+ CD8alpha–dendritic cell maturation and activation following viral infection of the central nervous system: implications for a role in T cell activation. Virology 327:8–15
97. Trifilo MJ, Montalto-Morrison C, Stiles LN, Hurst KR, Hardison JL, Manning JE, Masters PS, Lane TE (2004) CXC chemokine ligand 10 controls viral infection in the central nervous system: evidence for a role in innate immune response through recruitment and activation of natural killer cells. J Virol 78:585–594
98. Tsunoda I, Lane TE, Blackett J, Fujinami RS (2004) Distinct roles for IP-10/CXCL10 in three animal models, Theiler's virus infection, EAE, and MHV infection, for multiple sclerosis: implication of differing roles for IP-10. Mult Scler 10:26–34
99. Warmington KS, Boring L, Ruth JH, Sonstein J, Hogaboam CM, Curtis JL, Kunkel SL, Charo IR, Chensue SW (1999) Effect of C-C chemokine receptor 2 (CCR2) knockout on type-2 (schistosomal antigen-elicited) pulmonary granuloma formation: analysis of cellular recruitment and cytokine responses. Am J Pathol 154:1407–1416
100. Watanabe R, Wege H, ter Meulen V (1983) Adoptive transfer of EAE-like lesions from rats with coronavirus-induced demyelinating encephalomyelitis. Nature 305:150–153
101. Whiting D, Hsieh G, Yun JJ, Banerji A, Yao W, Fishbein MC, Belperio J, Strieter RM, Bonavida B, Ardehali A (2004) Chemokine monokine induced by IFN-gamma/CXC chemokine ligand 9 stimulates T lymphocyte proliferation and effector cytokine production. J Immunol 172:7417–7424
102. Widney DP, Hu Y, Foreman-Wykert AK, Bui KC, Nguyen TT, Lu B, Gerard C, Miller JF, Smith JB (2005) CXCR3 and its ligands participate in the host response to Bordetella bronchiseptica infection of the mouse respiratory tract but are not required for clearance of bacteria from the lung. Infect Immun 73:485–493
103. Williamson JS, Stohlman SA (1990) Effective clearance of mouse hepatitis virus from the central nervous system requires both CD4+ and CD8+ T cells. J Virol 64:4589–4592

104. Williamson JS, Sykes KC, Stohlman SA (1991) Characterization of brain-infiltrating mononuclear cells during infection with mouse hepatitis virus strain JHM. J Neuroimmunol 32:199–207
105. Wu GF, Dandekar AA, Pewe L, Perlman S (2000) CD4 and CD8 T cells have redundant but not identical roles in virus-induced demyelination. J Immunol 165:2278–2286
106. Xie JH, Nomura N, Lu M, Chen SL, Koch GE, Weng Y, Rosa R, Di Salvo J, Mudgett J, Peterson LB, Wicker LS, DeMartino JA (2003) Antibody-mediated blockade of the CXCR3 chemokine receptor results in diminished recruitment of T helper 1 cells into sites of inflammation. J Leukoc Biol 73:771–780
107. Xue S, Jaszewski A, Perlman S (1995) Identification of a CD4+ T cell epitope within the M protein of a neurotropic coronavirus. Virology 208:173–179
108. Zhang Y, Yoneyama H, Wang Y, Ishikawa S, Hashimoto S, Gao JL, Murphy P, Matsushima K (2004) Mobilization of dendritic cell precursors into the circulation by administration of MIP-1alpha in mice. J Natl Cancer Inst 96:201–209
109. Zhou Y, Kurihara T, Ryseck RP, Yang Y, Ryan C, Loy J, Warr G, Bravo R (1998) Impaired macrophage function and enhanced T cell-dependent immune response in mice lacking CCR5, the mouse homologue of the major HIV-1 coreceptor. J Immunol 160:4018–4025

Cytokine and Chemokine Networks: Pathways to Antiviral Defense

T. P. Salazar-Mather (✉) · K. L. Hokeness

Department of Molecular Microbiology and Immunology, Division of Biology and Medicine, Brown University, 69 Brown Street, Box G-B6, Providence, RI 02912, USA
Thais_Mather@brown.edu

1	Introduction	30
2	NK Cells and Antiviral Defenses	31
2.1	NK Cell Responses in MCMV Infection	32
2.2	NK Cell Inflammatory Responses in Liver During MCMV Infection	32
3	CCL3/MIP-1α: Primary Mediator of NK Cell Inflammation	34
3.1	MIP-1α and Antiviral Defenses: The Cytokine and Chemokine Networks	34
3.2	The Type 1 Interferons (IFN-α/β) Association	35
3.3	The CXCL9/Mig Association	36
4	CCL2/MCP-1: The First Link	36
4.1	Resident Macrophages: MCP-1 Producers	37
5	MCP-1 and Macrophage Recruitment	38
5.1	MCP-1 and Antiviral Defenses	38
6	Conclusions	38
References		40

Abstract The complex interplays between cytokines and chemokines are emerging as key communication signals in the shaping of innate and adaptive immune responses against foreign pathogens, including viruses. In particular, the virus-induced expression of cytokine and chemokine profiles drives the recruitment and activation of immune effector cells to sites of tissue infection. Under the conditions of infection with murine cytomegalovirus (MCMV), a herpesvirus with pathogenic potential, early immune functions are essential in the control of virus replication and virus-induced pathology. The coordinated MCMV-induced cytokine and chemokine responses promote effective natural killer (NK) cell recruitment and function, and ultimately MCMV clearance. The studies highlighted in this chapter illustrate in vivo pathways mediated by innate cytokines in regulating chemokine responses that are vital for localized antiviral defenses.

Abbreviations

MCMV	Murine cytomegalovirus
NK	Natural killer
MIP-1α	Macrophage inflammatory protein 1α
Mig	Monokine induced by interferon-γ
MCP-1	Monocyte chemoattractant protein-1
rIFN-α	Recombinant interferon-α

1
Introduction

The host response to microbial pathogens necessitates the integrated action of both the innate and adaptive arms of the immune system. Innate immunity is largely dependent on granulocytes, macrophages, dendritic cells, and natural killer (NK) cells, whereas adaptive immune responses require T and B lymphocytes. It is becoming increasingly evident that an effective immune response requires crosstalk among the various immune cells for linkage of innate and adaptive immunity. This intercellular network of communication signals is mediated in part by cytokine and chemokine responses generated against infectious agents, including viruses.

Cytokines constitute a group of low molecular weight soluble proteins that modulate various immune functions upon induction by various stimuli, such as bacterial or viral components [10–12, 32, 92]. Virtually all cells produce these proteins, including leukocytes and infected or activated nonimmune cells such as fibroblasts, endothelial cells, and a variety of tissue parenchymal cells [10, 11]. Cytokines control the magnitude and kinetics of immune responses by inducing or inhibiting the activation, proliferation, and/or differentiation of various target cells, and they also regulate the production of antibodies and other cytokines including chemokines [1, 11, 54].

Chemokines are small heparin-binding secreted cytokines that are functionally appearing to be more diverse than used to be thought. Housekeeping chemokines are generally constitutively expressed under physiological conditions, and they function in development and homeostasis [20, 56, 73, 81, 95, 104]. Inducible inflammatory chemokines function in the directed trafficking and localization of effector leukocytes within tissue compartments during inflammation, infection, and trauma [5, 58, 73, 82, 91, 95, 104]. There is considerable evidence highlighting the importance of chemokine-mediated inflammatory responses to pathogens as being crucial to survival during infections [18, 53–55, 57, 77, 78, 80, 83]. Additionally, it has become evident that infiltrating leukocytes may sometimes play a role in disease pathogenesis [18,

54, 55, 83, 98]. Nevertheless, as chemokines are central to the routing of key immune cells, they have emerged as key players in host defense mechanisms [54–58, 62, 80, 95, 104]. These proteins mediate their biological effects through selective interactions with seven-transmembrane G protein-coupled receptors on the surface of target cells [7, 9, 59, 74, 90]. Inflammatory chemokines are selective for a broad range of receptors. Nonetheless, in vivo studies have demonstrated specific functions for various chemokines [18, 19, 21, 25, 27, 37, 58, 80, 93].

Protective immunity to viruses is dependent on the activation and interplay between cytokines and chemokines to enhance or regulate innate or adaptive (or both) effector functions. Studies have demonstrated that the cytokine milieu induced by pathogens may determine the cellular constituents that get activated, and thus the nature of the immune response, by selectively inducing specific chemokines in infected tissue compartments [18, 37, 55, 57, 77, 78, 80]. The murine cytomegalovirus (MCMV) model of infection in the liver has been used to demonstrate the coordinated effects of activated cytokine and chemokine responses on the recruitment of NK cells to sites of infection to maintain early control of virus replication. This chapter presents a brief overview of the role of NK cells in antiviral defense, the molecular mechanisms regulating the innate cytokine and chemokine networks promoting NK cell inflammation into liver, and the conceivable role of these pathways in promoting downstream adaptive responses for effective antiviral defense.

2
NK Cells and Antiviral Defenses

NK cells are innate effector cells that respond quickly to a variety of pathogens before the onset of adaptive immunity [11, 96, 103]. These cells originate from bone marrow precursors and predominate in peripheral blood and spleen. However, they can be induced to traffic into other compartments including the liver during infection [77, 99]. Classical NK cells are $CD3^-$ and do not express rearranged antigen-specific receptors [11, 42, 71, 97, 103]. Instead, it is now widely accepted that NK cells express a complex repertoire of activating and major histocompatibility complex (MHC) class I-specific inhibitory receptors on their surfaces that interact with ligands on target cells [23, 101–103]. Engagement of activation receptors with ligands on infected cells permits NK cell-mediated killing and cytokine production, while the inhibitory receptors restrain NK cell activation [4, 23, 43, 101, 102]. The central role of NK cells as mediators of antiviral defenses has long been appreciated [11, 96].

Furthermore, viruses that evade immune detection by restricting the function of MHC class I T lymphocytes are more susceptible to NK cell-mediated protective responses [101–103]. These cells are quick to respond and can be activated to produce high levels of the cytokine interferon (IFN)-γ, as well as additional antiviral and immunoregulatory cytokines [11, 12]. NK cells have been demonstrated to mediate protection against a number of viral infections (reviewed in references [11, 12]), most notably is the extensive data documenting their importance in innate defenses against MCMV infection [6, 11, 15, 63, 64, 88].

2.1
NK Cell Responses in MCMV Infection

Resistance to MCMV infection is critically dependent on the activation of NK cells for early control of viral replication in target organs such as spleen and liver [11, 12, 14, 63, 77, 94], although T lymphocyte responses do get activated and contribute to viral clearance late in infection [35, 39, 69, 70]. The profound antiviral effects of NK cells against acute MCMV infection have been exemplified with a variety of experimental systems, including in vivo depletion of NK cells [14, 15, 63, 86], infection of beige mutant mice [66, 88], and most recently infection of mice deficient in NK cell, but not NKT or T cell, functions [50]. Together, these studies have demonstrated increased viral titers, liver pathology, and enhanced mortality upon elimination of functional NK cell responses. Conversely, resistance to MCMV infection has been demonstrated when NK cells were adoptively transferred into susceptible mice [16].

The mechanisms of NK cell-mediated defenses against MCMV infection in vivo have not been completely elucidated, although there is evidence that disparate NK cell responses are used in the spleen and liver for protection against MCMV infection. In the spleen, resistance seems to be mainly through perforin-dependent mechanisms, suggesting that NK cell-mediated cytotoxicity [94] and NK cell surface expression of an activating receptor [4, 23, 43, 101, 102], found on resistant strains of mice [4, 101], is required. In contrast, there is evidence that NK cell effector function in the liver is mediated through production of IFN-γ [52, 64, 77, 78, 94].

2.2
NK Cell Inflammatory Responses in Liver During MCMV Infection

The liver is a common target organ of MCMV infection [29, 61, 65, 87], and the rapid control of virus-induced disease is essential for survival [64, 65,

78, 80, 87]. As shown in Fig. 1a, the liver responds to MCMV infection by inducing a profound accumulation of inflammatory cells into the parenchyma that peaks between 48 and 72 h after infection of C57BL/6, 129SvEV, and T- and B cell-deficient C57BL/6-SCID mice [65, 77, 79]. Studies have identified NK cells as the major cellular constituents of the inflammatory foci [3, 22, 77]. As NK cells surround and sequester sites of MCMV antigen expression (Fig. 1b), it is highly conceivable that the inflammatory response limits the spread of infection to neighboring hepatocytes, thus minimizing virus-induced pathology. The precise effector mechanism used by inflammatory NK cells remains to be elucidated, although localization of IFN-γ within inflammatory sites ([77] and Sect.3) is critical to antiviral defense.

In vivo cell trafficking studies using fluorescently labeled bone marrow cells from either C57BL/6 or C57BL/6-SCID donor mice have demonstrated the rapid deployment and collective mobilization of NK cells between portal areas and central hepatic veins in MCMV-infected recipient mice [77]. Transfer studies using bone marrow donor cells from mice depleted of NK cell subsets using specific antibodies or from mice genetically deficient in NK cells and T lymphocytes demonstrated the accumulation of cells only in the liver sinusoids [77]. Thus, in vivo, NK cells are induced to migrate to sites in a pattern similar to the inflammatory foci observed in histological liver sections (see Fig. 1a).

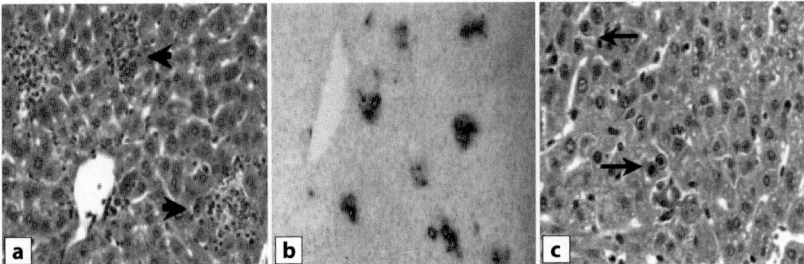

Fig. 1a–c Characterization of liver inflammatory foci during MCMV infection. a and b Paraffin-embedded or frozen livers sections were prepared from C57BL/6 mice infected with MCMV for 48 h and (a) stained with hematoxylin and eosin or (b) stained with immune serum antibodies to MCMV. Bound antibodies were detected with NBT/BCIP, followed by methyl green counterstain to highlight localization of inflammatory nuclei. *Arrowhead* denotes focus of inflammatory cells. c Paraffin-embedded liver sections were prepared from C57BL/6-MIP-1α deficient mice infected with MCMV for 48 h and stained with hematoxylin and eosin. *Arrow* denotes cytomegalic inclusion bodies

3
CCL3/MIP-1α: Primary Mediator of NK Cell Inflammation

To understand the key mechanisms governing the in vivo recruitment of NK cells to liver during MCMV infection, it is important to appreciate the chemokine expression profile. Of particular interest is the inflammatory chemokine CCL3 or macrophage inflammatory protein-1α (MIP-1α). Mice rendered genetically deficient in MIP-1α (MIP-1α knockouts) have been shown to exhibit reduced lung inflammation and delayed clearance of influenza virus when compared to control animals [19]. Moreover, MIP-1α promoted pulmonary inflammation and antiviral defense in a model of paramyxovirus infection [24]. During MCMV infection, MIP-1α messenger (m)RNA and protein can be detected in liver at times consistent with peak NK cell inflammation (48 h after infection) [77, 78]. Results obtained from in vivo cell trafficking studies demonstrated that the induction of NK cell inflammation in liver during MCMV infection was dependent on MIP-1α, as NK cell trafficking is dramatically impaired in MIP-1α knockout mice [77]. It is notable that monocyte and macrophage trafficking to liver is not affected in MIP-1α knockout mice, suggesting that although other chemokines are induced in these mice, MIP-1α responses are required for NK cell recruitment. Furthermore, MIP-1α knockout mice lacked detectable inflammatory foci in liver sections by histological evaluation, and displayed a profound increase in the number of cytomegalic inclusion bodies, or MCMV-infected cells (Fig. 1c) [77]. Flow cytometric analysis demonstrated that in the absence of MIP-1α function the absolute numbers of NK cells become significantly elevated in the blood but are dramatically reduced in the liver when compared to control mice [78]. These results imply that although NK cells get activated in response to infection, the communication signals directing their migration to tissue sites of virus replication are impaired in the absence of MIP-1α. Collectively, these studies define a prominent and unique role for MIP-1α in the initial influx of NK cells into the liver during MCMV infection.

3.1
MIP-1α and Antiviral Defenses: The Cytokine and Chemokine Networks

As discussed above, NK cells are an essential source of IFN-γ production that is required for early antiviral defense in liver. During MCMV infection, this cytokine is maximally elevated in spleen and serum within 40 h but subsides by 48 h after viral challenge [75, 78]. It has been established that an essential function of the MIP-1α-dependent NK cell inflammatory response is to sustain IFN-γ production in liver beyond the systemic kinetics of the cytokine, or further than 48 h [78]. MIP-1α knockout mice, with their inability to mount an effective NK cell inflammatory response, do not sustain sufficient levels of IFN-γ in the liver. The result is a profound elevation in spleen and liver viral titers followed by death on day 5 of MCMV infection. Interestingly, mice genetically deficient in interleukin (IL)-18 do not succumb to MCMV infection, although they are severely compromised in systemic, but not hepatic, IFN-γ responses [68]. Thus, MIP-1α functions promote viral resistance by mediating the recruitment of NK cells and the delivery of IFN-γ in a localized site of infection.

3.2
The Type 1 Interferons (IFN-α/β) Association

Early infection with MCMV induces production of multiple innate cytokines including the type 1 interferons, IFN-α/β [1, 11, 12]. These cytokines are potent activators of antiviral pathways [12, 36, 46, 84, 50] as well as mediators of multiple immunomodulatory functions, including induction of MHC class I expression, activation of NK cell cytotoxicity, and modulation of cytokines and cytokine receptors, including regulation of other type 1 interferon genes [12, 84]. IFN-α/β expression has also been shown to affect leukocyte trafficking [33, 38, 76, 79]. During MCMV infection, bone marrow-derived macrophages and NK cells have been shown to migrate to secondary sites in response to IFN-α/β production [76]. Recent studies have demonstrated production of IFN-α/β in MCMV-infected livers [79]. Histological analysis of liver sections in mice unable to respond to functions induced by IFN-α/β as a result of mutation in the receptor for the cytokines (IFN-α/βR knockouts) illustrated the lack of inflammatory foci but the presence of extensive virus-induced pathology in liver [79]. Moreover, IFN-α/βR knockout mice had reduced levels of MIP-1α protein in liver. Accordingly, IFN-α/βR knockout mice exhibit profound decreases in the accumulation of NK cells in liver. Furthermore, these mice exhibit mortality by day 5 of MCMV infection [79]. It is notable that NK cell accumulation is not significantly affected when uninfected MIP-1α knockout mice are treated with recombinant IFN-α (rIFN-α), indicating that IFN-α/β mediate immunoregulatory events upstream of MIP-1α.

In vivo cell trafficking studies demonstrated that leukocyte migration to the liver is dependent upon the effects of IFN-α/β, as only donor-derived fluorescent-labeled cells from immunocompetent—but not IFN-α/βR knockouts—accumulated extensively in liver [79]. Additionally, IFN-α/β mediated the recruitment of macrophage populations that were identified as a major source of MIP-1α production [79]. Altogether, these studies identify IFN-α/β as key mediators in the production of MIP-1α, and they define a cellular delivery mechanism driven by innate cytokines and chemokines for regulation of NK cell inflammation.

3.3
The CXCL9/Mig Association

One downstream consequence of the MIP-1α-dependent NK cell inflammatory response is induction of the IFN-γ-inducible chemokine CXCL9/monokine-induced by interferon (Mig), a potent T cell chemoattractant [2, 47, 49, 100]. Mig production is severely reduced in MIP-1α knockout mice when compared to control mice [78]. Furthermore, treatment of immunocompetent mice with immune serum against Mig resulted in highly significant increases in viral titers in both spleen and liver [78]. Consistent with results obtained using mice deficient in IFN-α/β and MIP-1α functions, Mig was required for survival, as neutralization of the chemokine led to death by day 5 of infection [78]. Studies have identified a prominent T cell response in liver by day 5 after MCMV challenge [28, 39]. It is therefore plausible that early expression of MIP-1α by MCMV-induced IFN-α/β recruits NK cells into the liver, and through localization of IFN-γ and subsequent Mig induction, these cytokine and chemokine networks provide an important link of innate and adaptive immune responses for overall antiviral defenses in tissue compartments. Ongoing studies in our laboratory are evaluating this likely scenario under the conditions of MCMV infection in the liver.

4
CCL2/MCP-1: The First Link

As discussed above, IFN-α/β clearly plays a role in promoting the recruitment of MIP-1α-producing macrophages into liver, but the primary molecular mechanisms guiding this process have only recently been examined during MCMV infection. Studies have identified CCL2, or monocyte chemoattractant protein-1 (MCP-1), as a key intermediate of IFN-α/β activity for regulation of inflammatory responses in liver [30]. MCP-1 production can be induced at this site as early as 24 h after MCMV infection. Furthermore, MCP-1 production precedes that of MIP-1α in a temporal fashion (Fig. 2) [30]. IFN-α/βR knockout mice show dramatic decreases in the levels of MCP-1 protein when compared to immunocompetent mice. In addition, the treatment of uninfected immunocompetent mice with rIFN-α results in a significant release of MCP-1 protein [30]. In vitro stimulation of naïve liver leukocytes obtained from immunocompetent mice with rIFN-α was shown to generate a dose-dependent induction of MCP-1. Together, these studies clearly establish that the induction of MCP-1 protein in liver is dependent on IFN-α/β-mediated functions.

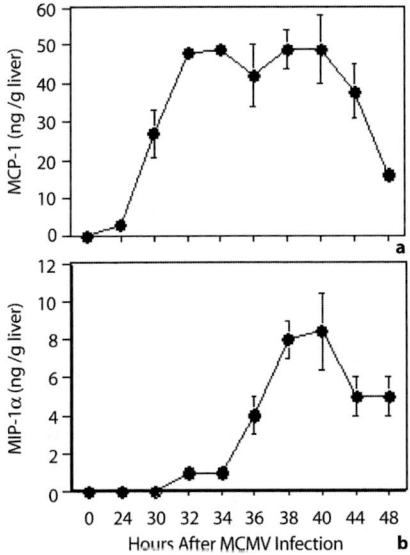

Fig. 2a, b Kinetics of MCP-1 and MIP-1α during MCMV infection in liver. Infected intraperitoneally with 5×10^4 plaque-forming units (pfu) MCMV were 129 mice. Livers were harvested from uninfected (0 h) or infected mice at the indicated time points. MCP-1 (**a**) and MIP-1α (**b**) protein levels in liver homogenates were determined by sandwich enzyme-linked immunosorbent assay (ELISA) [30]. The levels of detection were 0.08–0.2 and 0.02–0.05 ng/g liver for MCP-1 and MIP-1α, respectively. Data are the means±SE (n=3 mice tested individually for each time point). (Figure used with permission from [30]. Copyright 2005. The American Association of Immunologists)

4.1
Resident Macrophages: MCP-1 Producers

In multiple models of hepatic injury, resident macrophages have been shown to contribute to MCP-1 production [8, 44, 72]. The experiments highlighted in Sect. 4) strongly suggest that naïve liver leukocytes can be stimulated to release MCP-1 in the presence of IFN-α/β. Additional studies using enriched F4/80-positive and F4/80-negative cell populations—F4/80 being a mouse macrophage-restricted marker [45]—from uninfected immunocompetent mice demonstrated a clear induction of MCP-1 protein following stimulation with r-IFNα [30]. A similar induction of MCP-1 protein was observed with enriched F4/80-positive, but not F4/80-negative, cell populations from immunocompetent mice infected with MCMV for 24 h [30]. Thus, resident macrophages are early responders to the effects of IFN-α/β and are major producers of MCP-1 protein in liver.

5
MCP-1 and Macrophage Recruitment

It has been clearly established that MCP-1 effectively promotes the mobilization of inflammatory macrophages to sites of tissue damage [17, 26, 31, 51, 72] by preferential binding to the chemokine receptor CCR2 [13, 34, 40, 41, 67]. Recent studies have shown a dynamic impairment in liver macrophage and NK cell accumulation in mice deficient in MCP-1 (MCP-1 knockout) or CCR2 (CCR2 knockouts)—when compared to control mice—during infection with MCMV. Furthermore, MCP-1 and CCR2 knockout mice have decreased levels of both MIP-1α and IFN-γ proteins [30]. These results establish a central role for MCP-1 in promoting the recruitment of macrophages and NK cells. Moreover, they agree with previous observations that trafficking macrophages contribute to the initial release of MIP-1α, and subsequently the delivery of NK cell-derived IFN-γ in the liver [79, 80]. As CCR2 knockout mice displayed comparable responses, the results define MCP-1 as a key factor in initiating critical innate inflammatory events.

5.1
MCP-1 and Antiviral Defenses

It is clear from previous studies that MCP-1 is an important innate chemokine because it is uniquely necessary for monocyte and macrophage migration and the establishment of host defense against various pathogens [13, 18, 51, 31, 34, 40, 41, 85]. During MCMV infection, MCP-1 knockouts exhibit a marked elevation in spleen and liver viral titers by day 4 that remains prominent into day 5 of infection [30]. Comparable results were evident in CCR2 knockout mice. Increased viral burden was associated with increases in the circulating levels of the liver enzyme alanine aminotransferase, indicating liver damage. Accordingly, histological evaluation of liver sections prepared from uninfected control, MCP-1 and CCR2 knockout mice, did not show variability in appearance within the groups of mice (Fig. 3a–c). In contrast, on day 5 post-MCMV infection, MCP-1 or CCR2 knockout mice revealed large areas of necrosis as well as numerous cytomegalic inclusion bodies (Fig. 3e and f). Mortality in these mice coincided with virus-induced liver disease, as they succumbed to infection by day 5. This marked pathology was not evident in control mice. Instead, control mice displayed evidence of intermittent clusters of inflammatory foci, viral clearance, and were remarkably similar to the liver sections from the uninfected mice (Fig. 3a and d). These studies define a role for MCP-1, through interactions with CCR2, in promoting antiviral defense and protection from virus-induced liver disease.

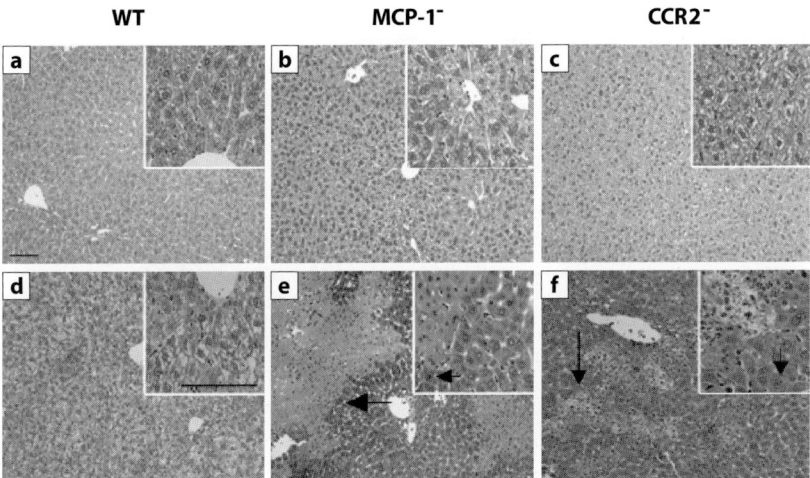

Fig. 3a–f Characterization of MCMV-induced liver damage in MCP-1- and CCR2-deficient mice. C57BL/6 (WT) (**a** and **d**) or mice genetically deficient in MCP-1 (MCP-1⁻) (**b** and **e**) or CCR2 (CCR2⁻) (**c** and **f**) were either uninfected (**a–c**) or infected with MCMV (5×10^4 PFU) for 5 days (**d–f**). Livers were harvested, paraffin was embedded, and they were sectioned for hematoxylin and eosin staining. *Bar* represents 100 μm. *Arrows* indicate necrotic lesions. *Arrows within insets* indicate cytomegalic inclusion bodies. Figure was used with permission from reference [30]. Copyright 2005. The American Association of Immunologists

6
Conclusions

The studies highlighted in this chapter define a network of cytokine and chemokine pathways that promote the activation, coordination, and shaping of the most effective immune response directed against a virus infection establishing itself in tissues. Specifically, the response elicits the migration of macrophages and NK cells by the selective induction of inflammatory chemokines (Fig. 4). The importance of chemokines to antiviral defense is underscored by the exploitation of the chemokine system by various human and mouse viruses, including herpesviruses, poxviruses, adenoviruses, and cytomegaloviruses [48, 53, 56, 60, 89]. Future in vivo studies dissecting the complex interactions between cytokines, chemokines, immune cell populations, and viruses will add to our understanding of immune regulation and perhaps the development of new therapeutic strategies for defense mechanisms against viral infections.

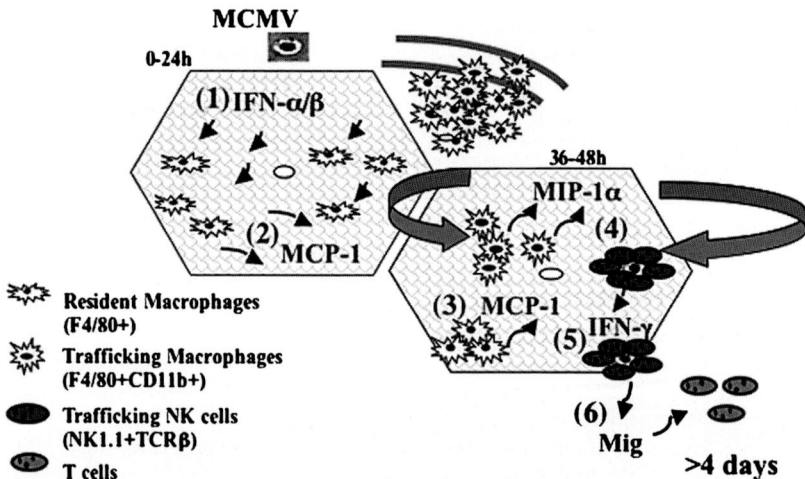

Fig. 4 Model of cytokine and chemokine interactions critical to antiviral defense during MCMV infection in liver. (*1*) The expression of the cytokine IFN-α/β is locally induced in response to MCMV challenge and (*2*) promotes the early release of MCP-1 from resident (F4/80+) macrophage populations. (*3*) MCP-1 initiates the recruitment of MIP-1α-producing macrophages from the periphery to the liver. (*4*) Subsequently, MIP-1α promotes the initial mobilization of NK cells from the periphery to the liver where they surround and sequester MCMV-infected cells to form characteristic clusters of inflammatory foci. (*5*) These events localize production of IFN-γ and (*6*) promote the induction of the IFN-γ-inducible chemokine Mig, a known potent chemoattractant of T lymphocytes. Together, these innate cytokine and chemokine interactions provide vital antiviral defenses in liver, and conceivably play a role in linkage of innate and adaptive immune responses

Acknowledgements Research in the authors' laboratory is supported by National Institute of Health Grant CA-102708.

References

1. Ahmed R, Biron CA (1998) Immunity to viruses. In: Paul WE (ed) Fundamental immunology, 4th edn. Lippincott-Raven, Philadelphia, pp 1295–1334
2. Amichay D, Gazzinelli RT, Karupiah G, Moench TR, Sher A, Farber JM (1996) Genes for chemokines mumig and crg-2 are induced in protozoan and viral infections in response to IFN-γ with patterns of tissue expression that suggest nonredundant roles in vivo. J Immunol 157:4511–4520
3. Andrews DM, Farrell HE, Densley EH, Scalzo AA, Shellam GR, Degli-Esposti MA (2001) NK1.1+ cells and murine cytomegalovirus infection: what happens in situ? J Immunol 166:1796–1803

4. Arase H, Mocarski ES, Campbell AE, Hill AB, Lanier LL (2002) Direct recognition of cytomegalovirus by activating and inhibitory NK cell receptors. Science 296:1323–1326
5. Baggiolini M (1998) Chemokines and leukocyte traffic. Nature 392:565–568
6. Bancroft GJ, Shellam GR, Chalmer JE (1981) Genetic influences on the augmentation of natural killer (NK) cells during murine cytomegalovirus infection: correlation with patterns of resistance. J Immunol 126:988–994
7. Bargatze RF, Butcher EC (1993) Rapid G protein-regulated activation event involved in lymphocyte binding to high endothelial venules. J Exp Med 178:367–372
8. Bautista AP (2002) Chronic alcohol intoxication primes Kupffer cells and endothelial cells for enhanced CC-chemokine production and concomitantly suppresses phagocytosis and chemotaxis. Front Biosci 7:117–121
9. Ben-Baruch A, Michiel DF, Oppenheim JJ (1995) Signals and receptors involved in recruitment of inflammatory cells. J Biol Chem 270:11703–11706
10. Biron CA, Cousens LP, Ruzek MC, Su HC, Salazar-Mather TP (1998) Early cytokine responses to viral infections and their roles in shaping endogenous cellular immunity. Adv Exp Med Biol 452:143–149
11. Biron CA, Nguyen KB, Pien GC, Cousens LP, Salazar-Mather TP (1999) Natural killer cells in antiviral defense: function and regulation by innate cytokines. Annu Rev Immunol 17:189–220
12. Biron CA, Dalod M, Salazar-Mather TP (2002) Innate immunity and viral infections. In: Kaufmann SHE, Sher A, Ahmed R (eds) Immunology of infectious diseases. ASM Press, Washington, pp 139–160
13. Boring L, Gosling J, Chensue SW, Kunkel SL, Farese SR Jr, Broxmeyer HE, Charo IF (1997) Impaired monocyte migration and reduced type 1 (Th1) cytokine responses in C-C chemokine receptor 2 knockout mice. J Clin Invest 100:255
14. Bukowski JF, Woda BA, Habu S, Okumura K, Welsh RM (1983) Natural killer cell depletion enhances virus synthesis and virus-induced hepatitis in vivo. J Immunol 131:1531–1538
15. Bukowski JF, Woda BA, Welsh RM (1984) Pathogenesis of murine cytomegalovirus infection in natural killer cell-depleted mice. J Virol 52:119–128
16. Bukowski JF, Warner JF, Dennert G, Welsh RM (1985) Adoptive transfer studies demonstrating the antiviral effect of natural killer cells in vivo. J Exp Med 161:40–52
17. Chae P, Im M, Gibson F, Jiang Y, Graves DT (2002) Mice lacking monocyte chemoattractant protein 1 have enhanced susceptibility to an interstitial polymicrobial infection due to impaired monocyte recruitment. Infect Immun 70:3164–3169
18. Chensue SW (2001) Molecular machinations: chemokine signals in host-pathogen interactions. Clin Microbiol Rev 14:821–835
19. Cook DN, Beck MA, Coffman TM, Kirby SL, Sheridan JF, Pragnell IB, Smithies O (1995) Requirement of MIP-1α for an inflammatory response to viral infection. Science 269:1583–1585
20. Cyster JG (1999) Chemokines and cell migration in secondary lymphoid organs. Science 286:2098–2102

21. Dieu MC, Vanbervliet B, Vicari A, Bridon JM, Oldham E, Ait-Yahia S, Briere F, Zlotnik A, Lebecque S, Caux C (1998) Selective recruitment of immature and mature dendritic cells by distinct chemokines expressed in different anatomic sites. J Exp Med 188:373–386
22. Dokun AO, Chu DT, Yang L, Bendelac AS, Yokoyama WM (2001) Analysis of in situ NK cell responses during viral infection. J Immunol 167:5286–5293
23. Dokun AO, Kim S, Smith HRC, Kang HS, Chu DT, Yokoyama WM (2001) Specific and nonspecific NK cell activation during virus infection. Nat Immunol 2:951–956
24. Domachowske JB, Bonville CA, Gao JL, Murphy PM, Easton AJ, Rosenberg HF (2000) The chemokine macrophage-inflammatory protein-1 alpha and its receptor CCR1 control pulmonary inflammation and antiviral host defense in paramyxovirus infection. J Immunol 165:2677–2682
25. Dufour JH, Dziejman M, Liu MT, Leung J, Lane TE, Luster AD (2002) IFN-γ-inducible protein 10 (IP-10;CXCL10)-deficient mice reveal a role for IP-10 in effector T cell generation and trafficking. J Immunol 168:3195–3204
26. Fuentes ME, Durham SK, Swerdel MR, Lewin AC, Barton DS, Megill JR, Bravo R, Lira S (1995) Controlled recruitment of monocytes and macrophages to specific organs through transgenic expression of monocyte chemoattractant protein-1. J Immunol 155:5769
27. Gao JL, Wynn TA, Chang Y, Lee EJ, Broxmeyer HE, Cooper S, Tiffany HL, Westphal H, Kwon-Chang J, Murphy P (1997) Impaired host defense, hematopoiesis, granulomatous inflammation and type1–type2 cytokine balance in mice lacking CC chemokine receptor 1. J Exp Med 185:1959–1968
28. Gold MC, Munks MW, Wagner M, McMahon CW, Kelly A, Kavanagh DG, Slifka MK, Koszinowski UH, Raulet DH, Hill AB (2004) Murine cytomegalovirus interference with antigen presentation has little effect on the size or the effector memory phenotype of the CD8 T cell response. J Immunol 172:6944–6953
29. Henson D, Smith RD, Gehrke J (1966) Non-fatal mouse cytomegalovirus hepatitis: combined morphologic virologic and immunologic observations. Am J Pathol 49:871–888
30. Hokeness KL, Kuziel WA, Biron CA, Salazar-Mather TP (2005) Monocyte chemoattractant protein-1 and CCR2 interactions are required for IFN-α/β-induced inflammatory responses and antiviral defense in liver. J Immunol 174:1549–1556
31. Huang D R, Wang J, Kivisakk P, Rollins BJ, Ransohoff RM (2001) Absence of monocyte chemoattractant protein 1 in mice leads to decreased local macrophage recruitment and antigen-specific T helper cell type 1 immune response in experimental autoimmune encephalomyelitis. J Exp Med 193:713
32. Ihle J (1995) Cytokine receptor signaling. Nature 377:591–594
33. Ishikawa R, Biron CA (1993) IFN induction and associated changes in splenic leukocyte distribution. J Immunol 150:3713–3727
34. Izikson L, Klein RS, Charo IF, Weiner HL, Luster AD (2000) Resistance to experimental autoimmune encephalomyelitis in mice lacking the CC chemokine receptor (CCR)2. J Exp Med 192:1075
35. Jonjic S, Mutter W, Wieland F, Reddehase MJ, Koszinowski UH (1989) Site-restricted persistent cytomegalovirus infection after selective long-term depletion of CD4+ T lymphocytes. J Exp Med 169:1199–1212

36. Katze MG, Gale Jr M (2002) Viruses and interferons: a fight for supremacy. Nat Immunol 2:675–687
37. Khan IA, Maclean JA, Lee F, Casciotti L, Dehaan E, Schwartzman JD, Luster AD (2000) IP-10 is critical for effector T cell trafficking and host survival in Toxoplasma gondii infection. Immunity 12:483–494
38. Korngold R, Blank KJ, Murasko DM (1983) Effect of interferon on thoracic duct lymphocyte output: induction with either polyI:C or vaccinia virus. J Immunol 130:2236–2243
39. Koszinowski UH, Del Val M, Reddehase MJ (1990) Cellular and molecular basis of the protective immune response to cytomegalovirus infection. Curr Top Microbiol Immunol 154:189–220
40. Kurihara T, Warr G, Loy J, Bravo R (1997) Defects in macrophage recruitment and host defense in mice lacking the CCR2 chemokine receptor. J Exp Med 186:1757–1762
41. Kuziel WA, Morgan SJ, Dawson TC, Griffin S, Smithies O, Ley K, Maeda N (1997) Severe reduction in leukocyte adhesion and monocyte extravasation in mice deficient in CC chemokine receptor 2. Proc Natl Acad Sci U S A 94:12053
42. Lanier LL, Cwirla S, Federspiel N, Phillips JH (1986) Human natural killer cells isolated from peripheral blood do not rearrange T cell antigen receptor β chain. J Exp Med 163:209–214
43. Lanier LL (2000) Turning on natural killer cells. J Exp Med 191:1259–1262
44. Leifeld L, Dumoulin FL, Purr I, Janberg K, Trautwein C, Wolff M, Manns MP, Sauerbruch T, Spengler U (2003) Early up-regulation of chemokine expression in fulminant hepatic failure. J Pathol 199:335–342
45. Lepay DA, Steinman RM, Nathan CF, Murray HW, Cohn ZA (1985) Liver macrophages in murine listeriosis. J Exp Med 161:1503–1512
46. Levy DE, Garcia-Sastre A (2001) The virus battles: IFN induction of the antiviral state and mechanisms of viral evasion. Cytokine Growth Factor Rev 12:143–156
47. Liu MT, Armstrong D, Hamilton TA, Lane TE (2001) Expression of Mig (monokine induced by interferon-γ) is important in T lymphocyte recruitment and host defense following viral infection of the central nervous system. J Immunol 166:1790–1795
48. Locata M, Murphy PM (1999) Chemokines and chemokine receptors: biology and clinical relevance in inflammation and AIDS. Annu Rev Med 50:425–440
49. Loetscher M, Gerber B, Loetscher P, Jones SA, Piali L, Clark-Lewis I, Baggiolini M, Moser B (1996) Chemokine receptor specific for IP10 and Mig: structure, function, and expression in activated T-lymphocytes. J Exp Med 184:963–969
50. Loh J, Chu DT, O'Guin AK, Yokoyama WM, Virgin IV HW (2005) Natural killer cells utilize both perforin and gamma interferon to regulate murine cytomegalovirus infection in the spleen and liver. J Virol 79:661–667
51. Lu B, Rutledge BJ, Gu L, Fiorillo J, Lukacs NW, Kunkel SL, North R, Gerard C, Rollins BJ (1998) Abnormalities in monocyte recruitment and cytokine expression in monocyte chemoattractant protein 1-deficient mice. J Exp Med 187:601
52. Lucin P, Pavic I, Polic B, Jonjic S, Koszinowski UH (1992) Gamma interferon-dependent clearance of cytomegalovirus infection in salivary glands. J Virol 66:1977–1984

53. Lusso P (2000) Chemokines and viruses: the dearest enemies. Virology 273:228–240
54. Luster AD (1998) Chemokines-chemotactic cytokines that mediate inflammation. N Engl J Med 338:436–445
55. Luster AD (2002) Role of chemokines in linking innate and adaptive immunity. Curr Opin Immunol 14:129–135
56. Mackay CR (2001) Chemokines: immunology's high impact factors. Nat Immunol 2:95–101
57. Matsukawa J, Hogaboam CM, Lukacs NW, Kunkel SL (2000) Chemokines and innate immunity. Rev Immunogenet 2:339–358
58. Moser B, Wolf M, Walz A, Loetscher P (2004) Chemokines: multiple levels of leukocyte migration and control. Trends Immunol 25:75–84
59. Murphy PM (1994) The molecular biology of leukocyte chemoattractant receptors. Annu Rev Immunol 12:593–633
60. Murphy PM (2001) Viral exploitation and subversion of the immune system through chemokine mimicry. Nat Immunol 2:116–122
61. Olver SD, Price P, Shellam GR (1994) Cytomegalovirus hepatitis: characterization of the inflammatory infiltrate in resistant and susceptible mice. Clin Exp Immunol 98:375–381
62. Oppenheim JJ, Zachariae COC, Mukaida N, Matsushima K (1991) Properties of the novel proinflammatory supergene "intercrine" cytokine family. Annu Rev Immunol 9:617–648
63. Orange JS, Wang B, Terhorst C, Biron CA (1995) Requirement for natural killer cell-produced interferon γ in defense against murine cytomegalovirus infection and enhancement of this pathway by interleukin 12 administration. J Exp Med 182:1045–1056
64. Orange JS, Biron CA (1996) An absolute and restricted requirement for IL-12 in natural killer cell IFN-γ production and antiviral defense. J Immunol 156:1138–1142
65. Orange JS, Salazar-Mather TP, Biron CA (1997) Mechanisms for virus-induced liver disease: a TNF-mediated pathology independent of NK and T cells during murine cytomegalovirus infection. J Virol 171:9248–9258
66. Papadimitriou JM, Shellam GR, Allan JE (1982) The effect of the beige mutation on the infection with murine cytomegalovirus: histopathologic studies. Am J Pathol 108:299–309
67. Peters W, Dupuis M, Charo IF (2000) A mechanism for the impaired IFN-γ production in C-C chemokine receptor 2 (CCR2) knockout mice: role of CCR2 in linking the innate and adaptive immune responses. J Immunol 165:7072–7077
68. Pien GC, Satoskar AR, Takeda K, Akira S, Biron CA (2000) Cutting edge: selective IL-18 requirements for induction of compartmental IFN-γ responses during viral infection. J Immunol 165:4787–4791
69. Quinnan GV, Manischewitz JE, Ennis FA (1980) Role of cytotoxic T lymphocytes in murine cytomegalovirus infection. J Gen Virol 47:503–508
70. Reddehase MJ, Mutter W, Munch K, Buhring HJ, Koszinowski UH (1987) CD8-positive T lymphocytes specific for murine cytomegalovirus immediate-early antigens mediate protective immunity. J Virol 61:3102–3108

71. Ritz J, Campen TJ, Schmidt RE, Royer HD, Hercend T, Hussey RE, Reinhertz EL (1985) Analysis of T-cell receptor gene rearrangement and expression in human natural killer clones. Science 228:1540–1543
72. Rollins BJ (1996) Monocyte chemoattractant protein 1: a potential regulator of monocyte recruitment in inflammatory disease. Mol Med Today 2:198
73. Rollins BJ (1997) Chemokines. Blood 90:909–928
74. Rossi D, Zlotnik A (2000) The biology of chemokines and their receptors. Annu Rev Immunol 18:621–648
75. Ruzek MC, Miller AH, Opal SM, Pearce BD, Biron CA (1997) Characterization of early cytokine responses and an interleukin (IL)-6-dependent pathway of endogenous glucocorticoid induction during murine cytomegalovirus infection. J Exp Med 185:1185–1192
76. Salazar-Mather TP, Biron CA (1996) NK cell trafficking and cytokine expression in splenic compartments after IFN induction and viral infection. J Immunol 157:3054–3064
77. Salazar-Mather TP, Orange JS, Biron CA (1998) Early murine cytomegalovirus (MCMV) infection induces liver natural killer (NK) cell inflammation and protection through macrophage inflammatory protein 1α (MIP-1α)-dependent pathways. J Exp Med 187:1–14
78. Salazar-Mather TP, Hamilton TA, Biron CA (2000) A chemokine-to-cytokine-chemokine cascade critical in antiviral defense. J Clin Invest 105:985–993
79. Salazar-Mather TP, Lewis CA, Biron CA (2002) Type I interferons regulate inflammatory cell trafficking and macrophage inflammatory protein 1α delivery to the liver. J Clin Invest 110:321–330
80. Salazar-Mather TP, Hokeness KL (2003) Calling in the troops: regulation of inflammatory cell trafficking through innate cytokine/chemokine networks. Viral Immunol 16:291
81. Sallusto F, Mackay CR, Lanzavecchia A (2000) The role of chemokine receptors in primary, effector, and memory immune responses. Annu Rev Immunol 18:593–620
82. Schall TJ, Bacon KB (1994) Chemokines, leukocyte trafficking, and inflammation. Curr Opin Immunol 6:865–873
83. Schluger NW, Rom WN (1997) Early response to infection: chemokines as mediators of inflammation. Curr Opin Immunol 9:504–508
84. Sen GC, Ransohoff RM (1993) Interferon-induced antiviral actions and their regulation. Adv Virus Res 42:57–59
85. Serbina NV, Kuziel W, Flavell R, Akira S, Rollins B, Pamer EG (2003) Sequential MyD88-independent and -dependent activation of innate immune responses to intracellular bacterial infection. Immunity 19:891–898
86. Shanley JD (1990) In vivo administration of monoclonal antibody to the NK1.1 antigen of natural killer cells: effect on acute murine cytomegalovirus infection. J Med Virol 30:58–60
87. Shanley JD, Biczak L, Forman SJ (1993) Acute murine cytomegalovirus infection induces lethal hepatitis. J Infect Dis 167:264–269
88. Shellam GR, Allan JE, Papadimitriou JM, Bancroft GJ (1981) Increased susceptibility to cytomegalovirus infection in beige mutant mice. Proc Natl Acad Sci USA 78:5104–5108

89. Smith GL (1996) Virus proteins that bind cytokines, chemokines or interferons. Curr Opin Immunol 8:467–471
90. Springer T (1994) Traffic signals for lymphocyte recirculation and leukocyte emigration: the multistep paradigm. Cell 76:301–314
91. Streiter RM, Standiford T, Huffnagle GB, Colletti LM, Lukacs NW, Kunkel SL (1996) "The good, the bad, and the ugly": The role of chemokines in models of human disease. J Immunol 156:3583–3586
92. Taniguchi T (1995) Cytokine receptor signaling through nonreceptor protein tyrosine kinases. Science 268:251–255
93. Taub DD, Conlon K, Lloyd AR, Oppenheim JJ, Kelvin DJ (1993) Preferential migration of activated CD4+ and CD8+ T cells in response to MIP-1α and MIP-1β. Science 260:355–358
94. Tay CH, Welsh RM (1997) Distinct organ-dependent mechanisms for the control of murine cytomegalovirus infection by natural killer cells. J Virol 71:267–275
95. Thelan M (2001) Dancing to the tune of chemokines. Nat Immunol 2:129 134
96. Trinchieri G (1989) Biology of natural killer cells. Adv Immunol 47:187–376
97. Tutt MM, Kuziel WA, Hackett J Jr, Bennett M, Tucker PW, Kumar V (1986) Murine natural killer cells do not express functional transcripts of the α, β or γ-chain genes of the T cell receptor. J Immunol 137:2998–3001
98. Wang J, Deng W Gong X, Su S (1998) Chemokines and their role in tumor cell growth and metastasis. J Immunol Methods 220:1–17
99. Wiltrout RH, Mathieson BJ, Talmadge JE, Reynolds CW, Zhang S, Herberman RB, Ortaldo JR (1984) Augmentation of organ-associated natural killer cell activity by biological response modifiers: isolation and characterization of large granular lymphocytes from the liver. J Exp Med 160:1431–1435
100. Wong P, Severns CW, Guyer NB, Wright TM (1994) A unique palindromic element mediates gamma interferon induction of mig gene expression. Mol Cell Biol 14:914–922
101. Yokoyama WM (1993) The Ly-49 and NKR-PI gene families encoding lectin-like receptors on natural killer cells: the NK gene complex. Annu Rev Immunol 11:613–644
102. Yokoyama WM (2000) Now you see it, now you don't. Nat Immunol 1:95–97
103. Yokoyama WM, Kim S, French AR (2004) The dynamic life of natural killer cells. Annu Rev Immunol 22:405–429
104. Zlotnik A, Yoshie O (2000) Chemokines: a new classification system and their role in immunity. Immunity 12:121–127

Herpes Simplex Virus and the Chemokines That Mediate the Inflammation

D. J. J. Carr[1,2] (✉) · L. Tomanek[1]

[1]Department of Ophthalmology, University of Oklahoma, DMEI 415, Health Sciences Center, 608 Stanton L. Young Blvd., Oklahoma City, OK 73104, USA
dan-carr@ouhsc.edu

[2]Department of Microbiology and Immunology, University of Oklahoma, Health Sciences Center, Oklahoma City, OK 73104, USA

1	Introduction	48
1.1	General Properties of Herpes Simplex Viruses	48
1.2	Herpes Simplex Virus Type 1	49
1.3	Herpes Simplex Virus Type 2	49
2	HSV-1 Infection of the Eye	50
2.1	Innate Immune Response to Ocular HSV-1 Infection	50
2.2	Chemokine Expression During the Innate Immune Response to Ocular HSV-1 Infection	51
2.3	Adaptive Immune Response to Ocular HSV-1 Infection	55
2.4	HSV-1 Latency in the Trigeminal Ganglion	55
2.5	Reactivation of HSV-1	57
3	HSV-2 Infection of the Genitalia	57
3.1	Immune Response to Genital HSV-2 Infection	57
3.2	Chemokines and HSV-2	58
4	Perspective	58
	References	59

Abstract Herpes simplex viruses (HSV) are highly pervasive pathogens in the human host with a seroconversion rate upwards of 60% worldwide. HSV type 1 (HSV-1) is associated with the disease herpetic stromal keratitis, the leading cause of infectious corneal blindness in the industrialized world. Individuals suffering from genital herpes associated with HSV type 2 (HSV-2) are found to be two- to threefold more susceptible in acquiring human immunodeficiency virus (HIV). The morbidity associated with these infections is principally due to the inflammatory response, the development of lesions, and scarring. Chemokines have become an important aspect in understanding the host immune response to microbial pathogens due in part to the timing of expression. In this paper, we will explore the current understanding of chemokine production as it relates to the orchestration of the immune response to HSV infection.

Abbreviations

HSV	Herpes simplex virus
PMN	Polymorphonuclear cell
NK	Natural killer
HSK	Herpetic stromal keratitis
IL	Interleukin
DC	Dendritic cell
Th1	T helper 1 cell
TG	Trigeminal ganglion
IFN	Interferon
TNF	Tumor necrosis factor
TLR	Toll-like receptor
VEGF	Vascular endothelial growth factor

1
Introduction

1.1
General Properties of Herpes Simplex Viruses

Herpes simplex virus type 1 (HSV-1) and type 2 (HSV-2) are neurotropic viruses that are members of the subfamily α-Herpesvirinae [42]. Both types of HSV are transmissible from person to person via infectious mucosal secretions that come in contact with mucosal epithelia that line surface apertures of the body [9, 42, 57]. Herpes simplex viruses can cause a variety of diseases including keratitis, cold sores, encephalitis, genital herpes, cutaneous herpes, and meningitis [12, 42]. HSV-1 and HSV-2 enter the epithelium of the host and initiate a lytic replicative cycle [18, 40–42, 57, 70]. HSV enters its target cell through a multistep process that includes envelope glycoproteins (g) that surround the viral particle [42, 64]. The initial interaction begins with the binding of gC and gB to heparin sulfate proteoglycans that are found on the surface of target cells [42, 64]. After the attachment of the viral particle to the host cell, another viral glycoprotein, gD, interacts with other host cell surface receptors, including herpesvirus entry mediator A, which is a tumor necrosis factor (TNF) receptor family member, and nectins, which allow for the fusion of the virion envelope to the cell's plasma membrane via gB, gD, gH, and gL [42, 64]. Local replication commences with transcription of viral lytic genes [18, 33, 40–42, 57, 64, 70]. Following a lytic replicative cycle, the virus enters sensory nerve endings in the basal aspect of the epithelium and undergoes retrograde transport to associated sensory ganglia [18, 42, 64, 70]. Within the sensory ganglia, HSV undergoes a second stage of lytic infection.

Depending on the extent of the infection, HSV may travel further to the central nervous system. Following acute infection of sensory ganglia, the virus establishes latency in a subpopulation of neurons [18, 42, 64, 70]. Periodic reactivation from latency during periods of stress or immune suppression results in the re-infection of the initial port of entry [18, 42, 70].

Clearance of the virus from the host is dependent on both the host's innate and adaptive immune responses. Polymorphonuclear cells (PMNs) are the first and most predominant cell type to infiltrate the area of infection, releasing a number of soluble factors including cytokines, chemokines, and tissue-degrading enzymes including matrix metalloproteinases [6, 22, 45, 96, 97]. Likewise, natural killer (NK) cells and subsequently, macrophages and T cells are recruited to the site of inflammation. Chemokine expression has become an interest in the scientific community as it relates to the immune response to infectious agents and the pathology that develops from this response.

1.2
Herpes Simplex Virus Type 1

The cornea is a transparent, avascular tissue composed of a surface epithelium, corneal stroma, and endothelium that covers the anterior portion of the eye [70]. It is the avascular nature of the cornea that preserves the visual axis, providing a translucent conduit for subsequent processing of an image by the lens and retina of the eye. However, experimental evidence suggests ocular HSV-1 can limit the visual axis through neovascularization and infiltration of leukocytes attracted to the site through the production of chemokines [103]. Experimental infection of the cornea initiates in the surface epithelium in the outermost squamous layer of cells. HSV-1 spreads from cell to cell in a polarized fashion to the next layer of cells, wing cells [70]. The virus is able to travel to the sensory nerve endings that can be found in the basal aspect of the epithelium [70].

One clinically significant disease that is caused by HSV-1 is herpetic stromal keratitis (HSK) an intense inflammatory response triggered by the viral infection of the corneal stroma [3, 45, 54]. If left untreated, the chronic inflammatory response leads to the formation of lesions, scarring, and eventually blindness.

1.3
Herpes Simplex Virus Type 2

HSV-2 is the causative agent of genital herpes of which approximately 500,000 new cases arise annually [33]. It has been estimated that 33% of the adult population is seropositive for this sexually transmitted disease, making HSV-2 the most common sexually transmitted pathogen worldwide [33, 73, 78, 92]. Genital herpes infection can result in complications including urinary retention and meningoencephalitis [33, 73, 78, 92]. Approximately 3,500 births in the United States are impacted by HSV-2 infection, which can lead to fatal infant encephalitis [18]. Even though a relatively large percentage of the population is seropositive for HSV-2, only a small percentage is subjected to these complications. Hormones have been implicated in the susceptibility to infection in the female host [86]. Specifically, mice exposed to progesterone are rendered more susceptible to infection [37] whereas estradiol-treated mice are found to be resistant to infection [27]. Although the role of ovarian sex hormones in susceptibility to genital HSV-2 infection is not completely defined, immune suppression [27], changes in the vaginal epithelial thickness [72], and modulation of a cell membrane receptor, nectin-1-δ [48], may all influence the infectious process.

One common denominator in the recruitment process of leukocytes into the inflamed HSV-infected tissue is the expression of chemokines. Although a necessary process in attracting immune effector cells required to control replication and spread of the virus, chemokine expression and the ensuing inflammatory response has detrimental consequences to the host, especially when considering the eye. Understanding the sequential expression of chemokines relative to ocular HSV-1 infection is pertinent to the development of a strategy that will ultimately control local inflammation and the collateral damage without rendering increased susceptibility to the host.

2
HSV-1 Infection of the Eye

2.1
Innate Immune Response to Ocular HSV-1 Infection

After initial infection of the virus into the cornea, an innate immune response is triggered to clear the pathogen. Toll-like receptors (TLR), a family of pattern-recognition molecules, are known to respond to pathogens and serve as early warning molecules that induce the expression of proinflammatory molecules [5]. Of the twelve TLR subtypes found in the mouse, TLR2 and TLR9 are expressed by corneal epithelium [36]. HSV-1 stimulates TLR2 by unknown means resulting in the activation of nuclear factor (NF)-κB and production of interleukin (IL)-6 [46]. HSV-1 which contains CpG motifs [106] is recognized by TLR9, resulting in the expression of type I interferon (IFN) [44]. In addition to the production of type I IFNs, the infected resident cells of the cornea as well as neighboring cells (most probably through TLR signaling and NF-κB activation) are known to release inflammatory cytokines including IL-1α, IL-6, and TNF-α [34, 88]. The absence or hindrance of these cytokines has been linked to a significant reduction in the incidence of HSK [6, 22, 101]. It is thought that IL-1α leads to the induction of IL-6 by resident corneal cells [6] that, in turn, elicit production of macrophage inflammatory protein-1α (CCL3) and -2 (CXCL2) [22] ultimately recruiting PMNs into the infected tissue. PMNs infiltrate the stroma underlying the infected epithelial cells, contributing to clearance of the virus and limiting viral dissemination within 24 h postinfection [6, 96, 97]. PMNs are thought to be a rich source of inducible nitric oxide synthase (iNOS) and TNF-α [13], the latter of which upregulates intercellular adhesion molecule (ICAM)-1 expression [69] facilitating the adherence of leukocytes to the endothelium [89]. The administration of monoclonal antibody to ICAM-1 [15] or use of ICAM-1-deficient mice [67] has not been found to diminish the infiltration of cells or the clinical course of herpetic disease following corneal infection. However, ICAM-1 does play a key role in preventing herpetic encephalitis [15, 67], suggesting pathways independent of ICAM-1 expression are involved initially in the recruitment of cells into the cornea, whereas controlling virus spread in the central nervous system involves ICAM-1 expression. After the initial infiltration of neutrophils, macrophages and NK cells infiltrate the area but PMNs remain the predominant cell type residing in the inflamed cornea up to the first 96 h postinfection [93].

2.2
Chemokine Expression During the Innate Immune Response to Ocular HSV-1 Infection

Evidence for the expression of chemokines in the cornea following HSV-1 infection was first described using endpoint polymerase chain reaction (PCR) in which KC (CXCL1), CXCL2, IFN-γ-inducible protein 10 (CXCL10), monocyte chemoattractant protein-1 (CCL2), MIP-1β (CCL4), and regulated upon activation, normal T cell expressed (CCL5) were observed [90]. While trauma to the cornea in the form of scarification induced the expression, continued expression of CCL2, CCL5, and CXCL10 were noted out to 72 h postinfection, whereas other chemokine messenger (m)RNA levels precipitously dropped in both BALB/c and outbred ICR mice [14, 90]. Of the chemokines noted above, CXCL1 and CXCL2 specifically target neutrophils principally through the receptor CXCR2 [11, 82, 99, 104]. Neutralization of CXCL2 with antibody leads to a reduction in polymorphonuclear neutrophil (PMN) infiltration into the cornea [54, 104]. Likewise, CXCR2 knockout mice infected with HSV-1 show a minimal infiltration of PMNs into the cornea [3]. Even with a reduction in PMN influx, HSK still develops in the CXCR2-deficient mice, which is thought to be due to an increase in IL-6 expression driven by elevated virus titers ultimately facilitating angiogenesis [3]. Although evidence suggests IL-6 can drive neovascularization through vascular endothelial growth factor (VEGF) in the cornea, the kinetics of expression of VEGF during the infectious process in this model suggests other dynamics are involved including T cells that are known to contribute to HSK [16, 83] and are a source of VEGF [63].

Whereas CXCL2 is thought to be induced by IL-6 [57], another CXC chemokine, CXCL10, has been found to be the only chemokine that is constitutively expressed in the cornea as determined by PCR [14, 90] and enzyme-linked immunosorbent assay (ELISA) [10]. CXCL10 levels rapidly rise in the cornea following HSV-1 infection, and neutralization of the chemokine dramatically reduces corneal edema and infiltrating cells [10]. The lone receptor for CXCL10 is CXCR3 expressed by NK cells, macrophages, dendritic cells (DCs), and activated T cells [21, 23, 47, 77, 94]. However, CXCR3 knockout mice ocularly infected with HSV-1 show a transient suppression of PMN ($Gr-1^+CD11b^+Mac-3^-$) recruitment into the cornea (D.J.J. Carr, unpublished observation), calling into question the role of CXCR3 and its ligands in PMN recruitment. However, other studies at different anatomical sites have described PMN infiltration as a result of CXCL10 expression [8, 105]. It is tempting to speculate that CXCL10 may upregulate CD11a on PMNs enhancing the adhesion to the endothelium as has been reported for Th1 cells [2] facilitating diapedesis into the stroma of the cornea. However, formal proof of this notion requires additional studies.

Of the CC chemokine ligands expressed during ocular HSV-1 infection, CCL2 is strongly expressed throughout the initial course of acute infection as measured by PCR [14, 90]. The role of CCL2 in the development of HSK may be peripheral to its effects on the recruitment of leukocytes into the cornea, since the administration of neutralizing antibody to CCL2 has no effect on the incidence of HSK in HSV-1-infected mice [99]. In contrast, the administration of anti-CCL3 antibody significantly reduces the severity of corneal opacity [99]. The kinetics of CCL3 expression suggest it is not a stimulus for the recruitment of leukocytes into the cornea until 7–10 days postinfection, a time that seems to correlate with the onset of HSK [99]. Consistent with this finding, mice deficient in CCL3 expression reportedly show little cellular infiltration in the cornea throughout the time course of infection with low to undetectable levels of T helper (Th)1 cytokines including IL-2 and IFN-γ [98] normally found during acute ocular infection [93]. Ironically, the CCL3 knockout mice clear the virus at the same time as wildtype control animals [99], which calls into question the mechanism of virus clearance. Since there is apparently little leukocyte infiltration, including PMNs, that is known to control HSV-1 replication in the eye [97]—with a paucity of $CD4^+$ T cells or IFN-γ present as well [99]—it is puzzling what mechanism(s) controls the virus.

Similar to CCL2, CCL5 is expressed throughout the course of acute HSV-1 infection [14]. CCL5, operating through its receptor CCR5, is a strong chemoattractant for T cells and NK cells [53, 80] but also influences PMN recruitment [71]. It is interesting to note that while HSV-1 tends to subvert immune activation, CCL5 is induced by HSV-1 through NF-κB and IFN regulatory factor 3 pathways [56].

The plethora of chemokines and proinflammatory cytokines produced in the cornea during the innate immune response (i.e., 0–5 days postinfection) may be generated from several sources. With the exception of CXCL10, the chemokines CXCL1, CXCL2, CXCL9, CCL3, and CCL5 are not constitutively expressed in the cornea (Fig. 1). Analysis by confocal microscopy has found the endothelial layer of the cornea expresses very modest amounts of the CXCL10 in uninfected mice (D.J.J. Carr, unpublished observation). Consistent with previous results [90], scarification of the cornea (a process typically employed

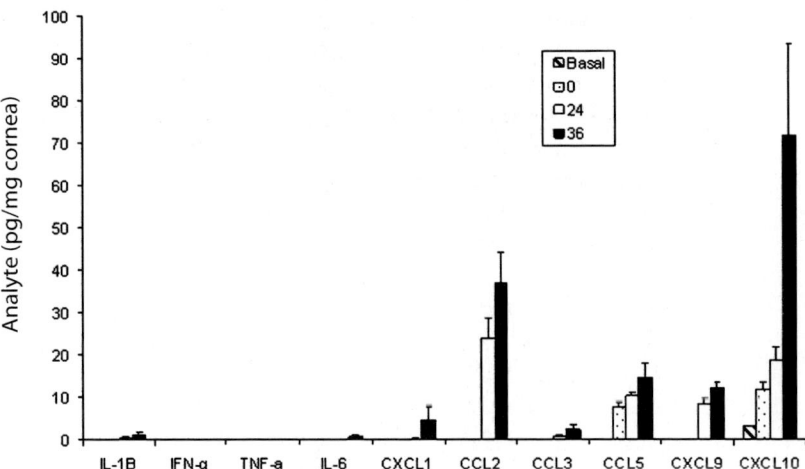

Fig. 1 Expression of inflammatory cytokines and chemokines in the cornea of HSV-1-infected mice. C57BL/6 female mice (n=6/timepoint) were left alone (*basal*) or scarified (*0*) and infected with HSV-1 (McKrae strain), 1,000 plaque-forming units (pfu)/eye. The mice were euthanized *24–36* h postinfection, perfused, and the cornea was removed and homogenized in a buffer containing a cocktail of protease inhibitors. The supernatant was clarified (10,000×g, 5 min) and assayed for cytokine/chemokine content by ELISA. *Bars* represents mean±SEM for each analyte under measure. CCL2 basal levels were not measured

to infect mice) alone elicits a rise in CCL3, CCL5, and CXCL10 expression (Fig. 1). Following infection, CXCL1, CCL2, CCL5, CXCL9, and CXCL10 are induced or upregulated within 36 h. Analysis of CCL5 and CXCL10 expression by confocal microscopy show two different patterns of expression. CCL5 is expressed in the epithelial layers of the eye colocalizing with HSV-1 antigen as well as within the stroma of the cornea (D.J.J. Carr, J. Ash, T. Lane, and W. Kuziel, submitted). By comparison, CXCL10 expression chiefly colocalizes with HSV-1 antigen expression in the epithelial layers of the cornea with punctate staining in the endothelium (D.J.J. Carr, unpublished observation). The expression profile of CCL5 and CXCL10 suggests the resident population generates most if not all of the CXCL10 within the first 24 h postinfection, whereas CCL5 is produced principally by resident cells but may also be provided by the infiltrating PMNs that are found within the stroma 24 h postinfection (D.J.J. Carr, J. Ash, T. Lane, and W. Kuziel, submitted). It is likely that as the infection

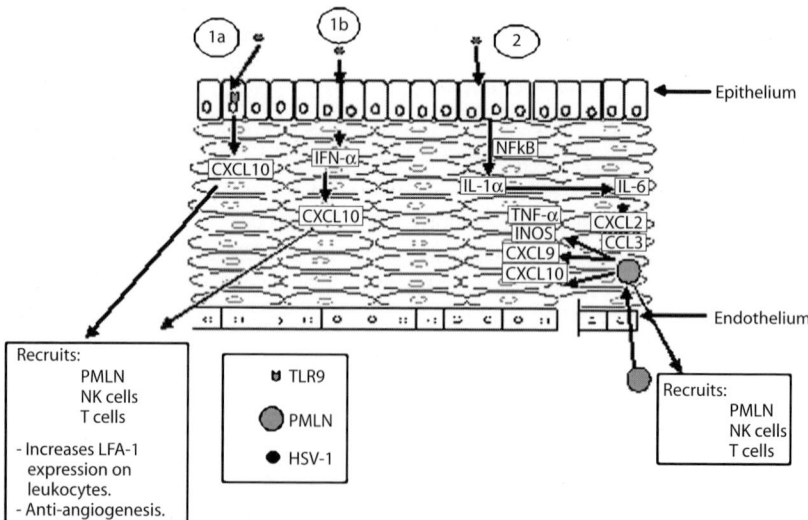

Fig. 2 Chemokine expression in the cornea following HSV-1 infection. Three different scenarios can operate in the production of chemokines within the cornea following ocular HSV-1 infection. In *1a*, HSV-1 DNA CpG motifs bind to the intracellular toll-like receptor (TLR)9 eliciting the production of CXCL10 through NF-κB activation. In *1b*, HSV-1 enters the epithelial cell and, following transcription, induces the production of IFN-α, which induces CXCL10 production. In *2*, HSV-1 activation of NF-κB stimulates IL-1α synthesis leading to IL-6 production, resulting in CXCL2 and CCL3 expression. These chemokines draw in PMNs and T cells. PMNs can secrete CXCL9 and CXCL10, which can recruit additional leukocytes including macrophages, DCs, NK cells, and T cells

spreads over the next several hours, chemokines generated including CCL2, CCL5, CXCL1, CXCL2, CXCL9, and CXCL10 are produced by multiple sources including the resident fibroblasts, epithelial, and endothelial cells as well as infiltrating PMNs, macrophages, NK cells, and DCs [11, 25, 82, 87, 100]. Collectively, the initial cascade of chemokine expression is complex but may be divided into two principal pathways involving CXCL10 and IL-6 (Fig. 2).

The delayed expression of CCL3 in the cornea is associated with a secondary wave of PMNs and some T cells into the stroma (day 10 postinfection) [99]. Since CCL3 targets monocytes, T cells, NK cells, basophils, eosinophils, DCs, and hematopoietic progenitors [11, 12, 82], it is currently unknown what events transpire to recruit the subsequent wave of cells. However, CCL3 is central to the effect since neutralizing this chemokine with antibody or suppressing expression with IL-10 reduces leukocyte recruitment into the cornea [99].

2.3
Adaptive Immune Response to Ocular HSV-1 Infection

Following the innate response to infection, preferential recruitment of Th1 $CD4^+$ T cells into the cornea is observed [35, 65]. Although it is currently unknown why there is a preferential recruitment of $CD4^+$ T cells into the cornea of HSV-1-infected mice, the expression of CXCR3 and CCR5 on activated T cells and the presence of CCL5 and CXCL9 in the cornea may influence the recruitment process [80, 81, 102]. The presence of $CD4^+$ T cells is crucial in controlling local virus replication and spread [7, 26] as well as the development of HSK [25, 58]. However, bystander activation of $CD4^+$ T cells in addition to virus antigen stimulation may also contribute to HSK development [24]. The continued expression of chemokines including CXCL2, CCL2, CCL3, CCL4, CCL5, and CXCL10 in the cornea would also provide the maintenance of leukocytes in the tissue recruited from the periphery and facilitate collateral damage to the cornea stroma [84]. Collectively, chemokines are instrumental in the initial trafficking of cells into the infected anterior segment of the eye as well as the development of HSK. Blocking their expression could preserve the visual axis, assuming local virus replication is controlled. A summary of chemokines expressed during the acute HSV-1 ocular infection is found in Table 1.

2.4
HSV-1 Latency in the Trigeminal Ganglion

After the successful infection of the cornea by HSV-1, a series of events occurs that can lead to a stable latent neuronal infection in the trigeminal ganglion

Table 1 Chemokine expression in the cornea during acute HSV-1 infection

Group	Name	Detection	Reference(s)
CXC	CXCL1	RT-PCR and ELISA	90, Fig. 1
	CXCL2	RT-PCR and ELISA	3, 6, 10, 22, 54, 90, 98, 104
	CXCL9	ELISA	10, Fig. 1
	CXCL10	RT-PCR and ELISA	10, 14, 90, Fig. 1
CC	CCL2	RT-PCR and ELISA	14, 90, 98, 99, Fig. 1
	CCL3	RT-PCR and ELISA	10, 22, 90, 98, 99, Fig. 1
	CCL5	RT-PCR and ELISA	10, 14, 90, Fig. 1

(TG) within 1–2 weeks postinfection [39, 41, 49]. Following an initial round of replication in the corneal epithelium, the virus is able to enhance its ability to access the axonal termini (via mechanisms that are not understood), and through retrograde axonal transport it enters the neuronal cell bodies in which another stage of lytic replication begins [49, 70]. After this brief replication cycle in the neuronal cell bodies, the lytic cycle genes are repressed and latency is established with minimal viral gene expression [49]. Infectious HSV-1 can consistently be detected in the TG out to approximately 10 days postinfection [12]. By day 30 postinfection, latency is established as defined by the lack of detectable infectious virions [12]. Even though infectious virions are not readily detected during latency, HSV-1 latency-associated transcripts (LATs) can be detected in the TG, and an associated local immune response is evident [28, 49]. With latency established, the immune system continually surveys the area with $CD8^+$ T cells as the principal cell type that is thought to prevent reactivation [39]. Along these lines, $CD8^+$ T cells are thought to control the infection through noncytolytic mechanisms using cytokines such as IFN-γ and TNF-α with minimal destruction to neurons [38, 50, 51, 95].

During latent infection, real time (RT)-PCR detection of CXCR3 and CCR5 expression has been reported [12]. Although unproven, it is likely these chemokine receptors are found on the $CD8^+$ T cells present in the TG during latency [29, 38]. Although ligands for CXCR3 including CXCL9 and CXCL10 have not been evaluated during latency, one ligand for CCR5, CCL5, has been detected [28]. Exposing latently infected mice to the potent antiviral compound acyclovir has been found to reduce CCL5 expression in the TG. Yet, the continued presence of CD8 cells suggests additional signals provide a stimulus for retainment of these effector cells within the tissue [29].

2.5
Reactivation of HSV-1

Due to a variety of environmental cues including UV light, stress, and immunosuppression, the virus is able to reactivate in the latently infected neurons of the TG. Through antegrade transport, the virus can again be detected in the corneal epithelium and stroma [68, 70]. The reactivation cycle can be repeated eliciting chronic and episodic immune activation, which leads to progressive scarring of the cornea resulting in decreased vision, glaucoma, iritis, cataract, and necrotizing retinitis [70]. While there is experimental evidence to suggest regulatory T cells may control ocular pathogenesis [91], how these cells impact on local chemokine expression is not understood.

3
HSV-2 Infection of the Genitalia
3.1
Immune Response to Genital HSV-2 Infection

During initial infection of the mucosa of the vagina with HSV-2, the virus begins to replicate in the epithelium, typically restricted to the epidermis or cervicovaginal epithelium [43]. The initial host response to infection includes the induction of type I IFNs (i.e., IFN-α species) through TLR9 recognition of HSV-2 CpG motifs [52]. The IFN-responsive pathway, double-stranded RNA-dependent protein kinase but not $2',5'$-oligoadenylate synthetases is essential for resistance to infection, as mice deficient in this pathway are highly susceptible to HSV-2-mediated mortality (D.J.J. Carr, L. Tomanek, R.H. Silverman, and B.R.G. Williams, manuscript in preparation). In addition to type I IFN production, IL-12, IL-15, IL-18, NK cells, and PMNs are important first lines of defense against HSV-2 replication and spread [1, 31, 59]. Current evidence suggests the resident populations of Langerhans cells [19] do not traffic to the inguinal/iliac lymph nodes with most migrating cells consisting of B lymphocytes [40]. T lymphocytes including γδ T cells are essential components of the adaptive immune response in controlling genital infection with HSV-2 [55, 60, 66, 73]. $CD4^+$ T cells produce the majority of IFN-γ in response to genital HSV-2 infection [32, 61]. Neutralization of IFN-γ leads to an increase in virus titer and a decrease in T cell recruitment into the vaginal tissue [61, 73]. B cell production of antibody is initiated in the draining lymph nodes and appears to have only a modest impact on HSV-2 titers, suggesting a limited role for B lymphocytes in the control of genital HSV-2 infection [17, 62, 75]. Manifestations of genital herpes include macules, papules, and vesicles resulting in the development of ulcers in the genital region [33]. Due to these ulcerations, other pathogens are able to enter into the vaginal mucosa. Recent studies have shown that patients who are infected with HSV-2 have a higher risk of contracting HIV-1 than patients who are HSV-2 seronegative with a two- to threefold increase in susceptibility [79].

3.2
Chemokines and HSV-2

The recruitment of leukocytes into the vaginal tissue following HSV-2 infection appears to include IFN-γ induction of the adhesion molecules ICAM-1 and vascular cell adhesion molecule 1 [76] since neutralizing IFN-γ diminishes lymphocyte infiltration into the infected tissue [74]. The expression of IFN-γ has also been associated with CCL5 production [30] found in the vagina following HSV-2 infection [4, 33]. The role of CCL5 expression in recruiting leukocytes into the infected tissue has not been described. However, plasmid DNA containing CCL5 has been found to enhance survival of HSV-2-infected mice [85]. Manipulating local expression of selective chemokines including CXCL2 and CCL3 using plasmid DNA suggests these chemokines may also play a significant role in protection for the host during genital virus infection by facilitating $CD4^+$ T cell immunity and elevating IFN-γ production by NK cells [20]. However, there are unresolved questions that remain as to those chemokines that initiate the inflammatory cascade as well as those that are critical for resistance to genital HSV-2.

4
Perspective

Chemokines are a significant group of soluble factors that contribute in the clearance of HSV-1 and HSV-2 pathogens from the host. Although necessary for an optimal immune response to the virus, chemokines initiate a frank inflammatory response that can result in a significant detrimental outcome to the host as it pertains to preservation of the visual axis. This chapter highlights the role of chemokines as they relate to the innate and adaptive immune response following ocular HSV-1 infection. Evidence suggests that curtailing expression of selective chemokines during HSV-1 infection of the eye may favor preservation of sight without consequences to controlling virus replication and spread. This observation suggests that while many chemokines are redundant in function and/or promiscuous in binding multiple receptors, selectivity in tissue expression of chemokines and targeting specific effector cells by those chemokines expressed in a given tissue may ultimately dictate the inflammatory response of the host and outcome of the infection. Understanding this process will prove beneficial in developing antiinflammatory therapies for individuals experiencing chronic HSV reactivation.

Acknowledgements The work was supported by a USPHS NIH grant, EY015566 and a Jules and Doris Stern RPB Research Professorship to DJJC.

References

1. Ashkar AA, Rosenthal KL (2003) Interleukin-15 and natural killer and NKT cells play a critical role in innate protection against genital herpes simplex virus type 2 infection. J Virol 77:10168–10171
2. Atarashi K, Hirata T, Matsumoto M, Kanemitsu N, Miyasaka M (2005) Rolling of Th1 cells via p-selectin glycoprotein 1 stimulates LFA-1-mediated cell binding to ICAM-1. J Immunol 174:1424–1432
3. Banerjee K, Biswas PS, Kim B, Lee S, Rouse BT (2004) CXCR2−/− mice show enhanced susceptibility to herpetic stromal keratitis: a role for IL-6-induced neovascularization. J Immunol 172:1237–1245
4. Benencia F, Gamba G, Cavalieri H, Courreges MC, Benedetti R, Villam SM, Massouh EJ (2003) Nitric oxide and HSV vaginal infection in BALB/c mice. Virology 309:75–84
5. Bhattacharjee R, Akira S (2005) Toll-like receptor signaling: emerging opportunities in human diseases and medicine. Curr Immunol Rev 1:81–90
6. Biswas P S, Banerjee K, Kim B, T Rouse B (2004) Mice transgenic for IL-1 receptor antagonist protein are resistant to herpetic stromal keratitis: possible role for IL-1 in herpetic stromal keratitis pathogenesis. J Immunol 172:3736–3744
7. Bouley DM, Kanangat S, Wire W, Rouse BT (1995) Characterization of herpes simplex virus type-1 infection and herpetic stromal keratitis development in IFN-γ knockout mice. J Immunol 155:3964–3971
8. Boztug K, Carson MJ, Pham-Mitchell N, Asensio VC, DeMartino J, Campbell IL (2002) Leukocyte infiltration, but not neurodegeneration, in the CNS of transgenic mice with astrocyte production of the CXC chemokine ligand 10. J Immunol 169:1505–1515
9. Brandt C R (2005) The role of viral and host genes in corneal infection with herpes simplex virus type 1. Exp Eye Res 80:607–621
10. Carr DJJ, Chodosh J, Ash J, Lane TE (2003) Effect of anti-CXCL10 monoclonal antibody on herpes simplex virus type 1 keratitis and retinal infection. J Virol 77:10037–10046
11. Chensue SW (2001) Molecular machinations: chemokine signals in host-pathogen interactions. Clin Microbiol Rev 14:821–835
12. Cook WJ, Kramer MF, Walker RM, Burwell TJ, Holman HA, Coen DM, Knipe DM (2004) Persistent expression of chemokine and chemokine receptor RNAs at primary and latent sites of herpes simplex virus I infection. Virol J 1:5
13. Daheshia M, Kanangat S, Rouse BT (1998) Production of key molecules by ocular neutrophils early after herpetic infection of the cornea. Exp Eye Res 67:619–624

14. Daigle J, Carr DJJ (1998) Androstenediol antagonizes herpes simplex virus type 1-induced encephalitis through the augmentation of type 1 IFN production. J Immunol 160:3060–3066
15. Dennis RF, Siemasko KF, Tang Q, Hendricks RL, Finnegan A (1994) Involvement of LFA-1 and ICAM-1 in the herpetic disease resulting from HSV-1 corneal infection. Curr Eye Res 14:55–62
16. Deshpande S, Zheng M, Lee S, Banerjee K, Gangappa S, Kumaraguru U, Rouse BT (2001) Bystander activation involving T lymphocytes in herpetic stromal keratitis. J Immunol 167:2902–2910
17. Dudley KL, Bourne N, Milligan GN (2000) Immune protection against HSV-2 in B-cell-deficient mice. Virology 270:454–463
18. Duerst R J, A Morrison L (2003) Innate immunity to herpes simplex virus type 2. Viral Immunol 16:475–490
19. Edwards JNT, Morris HB (1985) Langerhans cells and lymphocyte subsets in the female genital tract. Br J Obstet Gynaecol 92:974–982
20. Eo SK, Lee S, Chun S, Rouse BT (2001) Modulation of immunity against herpes simplex virus infection via mucosal genetic transfer of plasmid DNA encoding chemokines. J Virol 75:569–578
21. Farber JM (1997) Mig and IP-10. CXC chemokines that target lymphocytes. J Leukoc Biol 61:246–257
22. Fenton R R, Molesworth-Kenyon S, E Oakes J, N Lausch R (2002) Linkage of IL-6 with neutrophil chemoattractant expression in virus-induced ocular inflammation. Invest Ophthalmol 43:737–743
23. Foley JF, Yu R Solow CR, Yacobucci M, Peden KW, M Farber J (2005) Roles for CXC chemokine ligands 10 and 11 in recruiting CD4+ T cells to HIV-1-infected monocyte-derived macrophages, dendritic cells, and lymph nodes. J Immunol 174:4892–4900
24. Gangappa S, Babu JS, Thomas J, Daheshia M, Rouse BT (1998) Virus-induced immunoinflammatory lesions in the absence of viral antigen recognition. J Immunol 161:4289–4300
25. Gasperini S, Marchi M, Calzetti F, Laudanna C, Vicentini L, Olsen H, Murphy M, Liao F, Farber J, Cassatella MA (1999) Gene expression and production of the monokine induced by IFN-γ (MIG), IFN-inducible T cell α chemoattractant (I-TAC), and IFN-γ-inducible protein-10 (IP-10) chemokines by human neutrophils. J Immunol 162:4928–4937
26. Ghiasi H, Cai S, Perng GC, Nesburn AB, Wechsler SL (2000) Both CD4+ and CD8+ T cells are involved in protection against HSV-1 induced corneal scarring. Br J Ophthalmol 84:408–412
27. Gillgrass AE, Fernandez SA, Rosenthal KL, Kaushic C (2005) Estradiol regulates susceptibility following primary exposure to genital herpes simplex virus type 2, while progesterone induces inflammation. J Virol 79:3107–3116
28. Halford WP, Gebhardt BM, Carr DJJ (1996) Persistent cytokine expression in trigeminal ganglion latently infected with herpes simplex virus type 1. J Immunol 157:3542–3549
29. Halford WP, Gebhardt BM, Carr DJJ (1997) Acyclovir blocks cytokine gene expression in trigeminal ganglia latently infected with herpes simplex virus type 1. Virology 238:53–63

30. Harandi AM, Svennerholm B, Holmgren J, Eriksson K (2001) Protective vaccination against genital herpes simplex virus type (HSV-2) infection in mice is associated with a rapid induction of local IFN-gamma-dependent RANTES production following a vaginal viral challenge. Am J Reprod Immunol 46:420–424
31. Harandi AM, Svennerholm B, Holmgren J, Eriksson K (2001) Interleukin-12 (IL-12) and IL-18 are important in innate defense against genital herpes simplex virus type 2 infection in mice but are not required for the development of acquired gamma interferon-mediated protective immunity. J Virol 75:6705–6709
32. Harandi AM, Svennerholm B, Holmgren J, Eriksson K (2001) Differential roles of B cells and IFN-γ-secreting CD4+ T cells in innate and adaptive immune control of genital herpes simplex virus type 2 infection in mice. J Gen Virol 82:845–853
33. Harle P, Noisakran S, Carr DJJ (2001) The application of a plasmid DNA encoding IFN-α1 postinfection enhances cumulative survival of herpes simplex virus type 2 vaginally infected mice. J Immunol 166:1803–1812
34. He J, Ichimura H, Iida T, Minami M, Kobayashi K, Kita M, Sotozono C, Tagawa YI, Iwakura Y, Imanishi J (1999) Kinetics of cytokine production in the cornea and trigeminal ganglion of C57BL/6 mice after corneal HSV-1 infection. J Interferon Cytokine Res 19:609–615
35. Hendricks RL, Janowicz M, Tumpey TM (1992) Critical role of corneal Langerhans cells in the CD4+ mediated but not CD8+ mediated immunopathology in herpes simplex virus-1 infected corneas. J Immunol 148:2522–2529
36. Johnson AC, Heinzel FP, Diaconu E, Sun Y, Hise AG, Golenbock D, Lass JH, Pearlman E (2005) Activation of toll-like receptor (TLR)2, TLR4, and TLR9 in the mammalian cornea induces MyD88-dependent corneal inflammation. Invest Ophthalmol Vis Sci 46:589–595
37. Kaushic C, Ashkar AA, Reid LA, Rosenthal KL (2003) Progesterone increases susceptibility and decreases immune responses to genital herpes infection. J Virol 77:4558–4565
38. Khanna KM, Bonneau RH, Kinchington PR, Hendricks RL (2003) Herpes simplex virus-specific memory CD8+ T cells are selectively activated and retained in latently infected sensory ganglia. Immunity 18:593–603
39. Khanna K M, J Lepisto A, Decman V, L Hendricks R (2004) Immune control of herpes simplex virus during latency. Curr Opin Immunol 16:463–469
40. King NJC, Parr EL, Parr MB (1998) Migration of lymphoid cells from vaginal epithelium to iliac lymph nodes in relation to vaginal infection by herpes simplex virus type 2. J Immunol 160:1173–1180
41. Kodukula P, Liu T, Rooijen NV, Jager MJ, Hendricks RL (1999) Macrophage control of herpes simplex virus type 1 replication in the peripheral nervous system. J Immunol 162:2895–2905
42. Koelle DM, Corey L (2003) Recent progress in herpes simplex virus immunobiology and vaccine research. Clin Microbiol Rev 16:96–113
43. Koelle D M, C Gonzalez J, S Johnson A (2005) Homing in on the cellular immune response to HSV-2 in humans. Am J Reprod Immunol 53:172–181
44. Krug A, Luker GD, Barchet W, Leib DA, Akira S, Colonna M (2004) Herpes simplex virus type 1 activates murine natural interferon-producing cells through toll-like receptor 9. Blood 103:1433–1437

45. Kumaraguru U, Davis I, Rouse BT (1999) Chemokines and ocular pathology caused by corneal infection with herpes simplex virus. J NeuroVirol 5:42–47
46. Kurt-Jones EA, Chan M, Zhou S, Wang J, Reed G, Bronson R, Arnold MM, Knipe DM, Finberg RW (2004) Herpes simplex virus 1 interaction with toll-like receptor 2 contributes to lethal encephalitis. Proc Natl Acad Sci USA 101:1315–1320
47. Lang A, Nikolich-Zugich J (2005) Development and migration of protective CD8+ T cells into the nervous system following ocular herpes simplex virus-1 infection. J Immunol 174:2919–2925
48. Linehan MM, Richman S, Krummenacher C, Eisenberg RJ, Cohen GH, Iwasaki A (2004) In vivo role of nectin-1 in entry of herpes simplex virus type 1 (HSV-1) and HSV-2 through the vaginal mucosa. J Virol 78:2530–2536
49. Liu T, Tang Q, L Hendricks R (1996) Inflammatory infiltration of the trigeminal ganglion after herpes simplex virus type 1 corneal infection. J Virol 70:264–271
50. Liu T, Khanna KM, Chen XP, Fink DJ, Hendricks RL (2000) CD8+ T cells can block herpes simplex virus type 1 (HSV-1) reactivation from latency in sensory neurons. J Exp Med 191:1459–1466
51. Liu T, Khanna KM, Carriere BN, Hendricks RL (2001) Gamma interferon can prevent herpes simplex virus type 1 reactivation from latency in sensory neurons. J Virol 75:11178–11184
52. Lund J, Sato A, Akira S, Medzhitov R, Iwasaki A (2003) Toll-like receptor 9-mediated recognition of herpes simplex virus-2 by plasmacytoid dendritic cells. J Exp Med 198:513–520
53. Mack M, Cihak J, Simonis C, Luckow B, Proudfoot AEI, Plachy J, Bruhl H, Frink M, J Anders H, Vielhauer V, Pfirstinger J, Stangassinger M, Schlondorff D (2001) Expression and characterization of the chemokine receptors CCR2 and CCR5 in mice. J Immunol 166:4697–4704
54. Maertzdorf J, Osterhaus AD, Verjans GM (2002) IL-17 expression in human herpetic stromal keratitis: modulatory effects on chemokine production by corneal fibroblasts. J Immunol 169:5897–5903
55. McDermott MR, Goldsmith CH, Rosenthal KL, Brais LJ (1989) T lymphocytes in genital lymph nodes protect mice from intravaginal infection with herpes simplex virus type 2. J Infect Dis 159:460–466
56. Melchjorsen J, R Paludan S (2003) Induction of RANTES/CCL5 by herpes simplex virus is regulated by nuclear factor κB and interferon regulatory factor 3. J Gen Virol 84:2491–2495
57. Melchjorsen J, Pedersen FS, Mogensen SC, Paludan SR (2002) Herpes simplex virus selectively induces expression of the CC chemokine RANTES/CCL5 in macrophages through a mechanism dependent on PKR and ICP0. J Virol 76:2780–2788
58. Mercadal CM, Bouley DM, DeStephano D, Rouse BT (1993) Herpetic stromal keratitis in the reconstituted SCID mouse model. J Virol 67:3404–3408
59. Milligan GN (1999) Neutrophils aid in protection of the vaginal mucosae of immune mice against challenge with herpes simplex virus type 2. J Virol 73:6380–6386

60. Milligan GN, Bernstein DI (1995a) Analysis of herpes simplex virus-specific T cells in the murine female genital tract following genital infection with herpes simplex virus type 2. Virology 212:481–489
61. Milligan GN, Bernstein DI (1997) Interferon-γ enhances resolution of herpes simplex virus type 2 infection of the murine genital tract. Virology 229:259–268
62. Milligan GN, Bernstein DI (1995b) Generation of humoral immune responses against herpes simplex virus type 2 in the murine female genital tract. Virology 206:234–241
63. Mor F, Quintana FJ, Cohen IR (2004) Angiogenesis-inflammation cross-talk: vascular endothelial growth factor is secreted by activated T cells and induces Th1 polarization. J Immunol 172:4618–4623
64. Mossman K L, F Macgregor P, J Rozmus J, B Goryachev A, M Edwards A, R Smiley J (2001) Herpes simplex virus triggers and then disarms a host antiviral response. J Virol 75:750–758
65. Niemialtowski MG, Rouse BT (1992) Predominance of Th1 cells in ocular tissues during herpetic stromal keratitis. J Immunol 149:3035–3039
66. Nishimura H, Yahima T, Kagimoto Y, Ohata M, Watase T, Kishihara K, Goshima F, Nishiyama Y, Yoshikai Y (2004) Intraepithelial γδ T cells may bridge a gap between innate immunity and acquired immunity to herpes simplex virus type 2. J Virol 78:4927–4930
67. Noisakran S, Härle P, Carr DJJ (2001) ICAM-1 is required for resistance to herpes simplex virus type 1 but no interferon-α1 transgene efficacy. Virology 283:69–77
68. Noisakran S, P Halford W, Veress L, JJ Carr D (1998) Role of the hypothalamic pituitary adrenal axis and IL-6 in stress-induced reactivation of latent herpes simplex virus type 1. J Immunol 160:5441–5447
69. Norris DA (1990) Cytokine modulation of adhesion molecules in the regulation of immunologic cytotoxicity of epidermal targets. J Invest Dermatol 95:111S–120S
70. Ohara P T, S Chin M, H LaVail J (2000) The spread of herpes simplex virus type 1 from trigeminal neurons to the murine cornea: an immunoelectron microscopy Study. J Virol 74:4776–4786
71. Pan ZZ, Parkyn L, Ray A, Ray P (2000) Inducible lung-specific expression of RANTES: preferential recruitment of neutrophils. Am J Physiol Lung Cell Mol Physiol 279:L658–L666
72. Parr MB, Kepple L, McDermott MR, Drew MD, Bozzola JJ, Parr EL (1994) A mouse model for studies of mucosal immunity to vaginal infection by herpes simplex virus type 2. Lab Invest 70:369–380
73. Parr M B, L Parr E (1998) Mucosal immunity to herpes simplex virus type 2 infections in the mouse vagina is impaired by in vivo depletion of T lymphocytes. J Virol 72:2677–2685
74. Parr MB, Parr EL (1999) The role of gamma interferon in immune resistance to vaginal infection by herpes simplex virus type 2 in mice. Virology 258:282–294
75. Parr MB, Harriman GR, Parr EL (1998) Immunity to vaginal HSV-2 infection in immunoglobulin A knockout mice. Immunology 95:208–213
76. Parr MB, Parr EL (2000) Interferon-γ up-regulates intercellular adhesion molecule-1 and vascular adhesion molecule-1 and recruits lymphocytes into the vagina of immune mice challenged with herpes simplex virus type 2. Immunology 99:540–545

77. Piali L, Weber C, LaRosa G, Mackay CR, Springer TA, Clark-Lewis I, Moser B (1998) The chemokine receptor CXCR3 mediates rapid and shearing resistant adhesion-induction of effector T lymphocytes by the chemokines IP10 and Mig. Eur J Immunol 28:961–972
78. Posavad C M, I Huang M, Barcy S, M Koelle D, Corey L (2000) Long term persistence of herpes simplex virus-specific CD8+ CTL in persons with frequently recurring genital herpes. J Immunol 165:1146–1152
79. Posavad C M, M Koelle D, F Shaughnessy M, Corey L (1997) Severe genital herpes infections in HIV-infected individuals with impaired herpes simplex virus-specific CD8+ cytotoxic T lymphocyte responses. Proc Natl Acad Sci USA 94:10289–10294
80. Qin S, Rottman JB, Myers P, Kassam N, Weinblatt M, Loetscher M, Ko AE, Moser B, Mackay CR (1998) The chemokine receptors CXCR3 and CCR5 mark subsets of T cells associated with certain inflammatory reactions. J Clin Invest 101:746–754
81. Rabin RL, Alston MA, Sircus JC, Knollmann-Ritschel B, Moratz C, Ngo D, Farber JM (2003) CXCR3 is induced early on the pathway of CD4+ T cell differentiation and bridges central and peripheral functions. J Immunol 171:2812–2824
82. Rollins BJ (1997) Chemokines. Blood 90:909–928
83. Russell RG, Nasisse MP, Larsen S, Rouse BT (1984) Role of T-lymphocytes in the pathogenesis of herpetic stromal keratitis. Invest Ophthalmol Vis Sci 25:938–944
84. Seo SK, Park HY, Choi JH, Kim WY, Kim YH, Jung HW, Kwon B, Lee HW, Kwon BS (2003) Blocking 4-1BB/4-1BB ligand interactions prevents herpetic stromal keratitis. J Immunol 171:576–583
85. Sin J, Kim JJ, Pachuk C, Satishchandran C, Weiner DB (2000) DNA vaccines encoding interleukin-8 and RANTES enhance antigen-Specific Th1-Type CD4+ T-cell-mediated protective immunity against Herpes simplex virus type 2 in vivo. J Virol 74:11173–11180
86. Sonnex G (1998) Influence of ovarian hormones on urogenital infection. Sex Transm Infect 74:11–19
87. Sonoda K-H, Sasa Y, Qiao H, Tsutsumi C, Hisatomi T, Komiyama S, Kubota T, Sakamoto T, I Kawano Y, Ishibashi T (2003) Immunoregulatory role of ocular macrophages: the macrophage produce RANTES to suppress experimental autoimmune uveitis. J Immunol 171:2652–2659
88. Staats HF, Lausch RN (1993) Cytokine expression in vivo during murine herpetic stromal keratis. J Immunol 151:277–283
89. Stewart MR, Cabanas C, Hogg N (1996) T cell adhesion to intercellular adhesion molecule-1 (ICAM-1) is controlled by cell spreading and the activation of integrin LFA-1. J Immunol 156:1810–1817
90. Su YH, Yan XT, Oakes JE, Lausch RN (1996) Protective antibody therapy is associated with reduced chemokine transcripts in herpes simplex virus type 1 corneal infection. J Virol 70:1277–1281
91. Suvas S, Azkur AK, Kim BS, Kumaraguru U, Rouse BT (2004) CD4+CD25+ T cells control the severity of viral immunoinflammatory lesions. J Immunol 172:4123–4132
92. Svensson A, Nordstrom I, Sun JB, Eriksson K (2005) Protective immunity to genital herpes simplex virus type 2 infection is mediated by T-bet. J Immunol 174:6266–6273

93. Tang Q, Chen W, Hendricks RL (1997) Proinflammatory functions of IL-2 in herpes simplex virus corneal infection. J Immunol 158:1275–1283
94. Taub DD, Lloyd AR, Conlon K, Wang JM, Ortaldo JR, Harada A, Matsushima K, Kelvin DJ, Oppenheim JJ (1993) Recombinant human-interferon-inducible protein 10 is a chemoattractant for human monocytes and T lymphocytes and promotes T cell adhesion and endothelial cells. J Exp Med 177:1809–1814
95. Theil D, Derfuss T, Paripovic I, Herberger S, Meinl E, Schueler O, Strupp M, Arbusow V, Brandt T (2003) Latent Herpesvirus Infection in Human Trigeminal Ganglia Causes Chronic Immune Response. Am J Pathol 163:2179–2184
96. Thomas J, Gangappa S, Kanangat S, T Rouse B (1997) On the essential involvement of neutrophils in the immunopathology disease. J Immunol 158:1383–1391
97. Tumpey T M, Chen S, E Oakes J, N Lausch R (1996) Neutrophil-mediated suppression of virus replication after herpes simplex virus type 1 infection of the murine cornea. J Virol 70:898–904
98. Tumpey TM, Cheng H, Cook DN, Smithies O, Oakes JE, Lausch RN (1998) Absence of macrophage inflammatory protein-1α prevents the development of blinding herpes stromal keratitis. J Virol 72:3705–3710
99. Tumpey TM, Cheng H, Yan X, Oakes JE, Lausch RN (1998) Chemokine synthesis in the HSV-1-infected cornea and its suppression by interleukin-10. J Leukoc Biol 63:486–492
100. Van Damme J, Decock B, Bertini R, Conings R, Lenaerts JP, Put W, Opdenakker G, Mantovani A (1991) Production and identification of natural monocyte chemotactic protein from virally infected murine fibroblasts. Relationship with the product of the mouse competence (JE) gene. Eur J Biochem 199:223–229
101. Wasmuth S, Bauer D, Yang Y, P Steuhl K, Heiligenhaus A (2003) Topical treatment with antisense oligonucleotides targeting tumor necrosis factor-α in herpetic stromal keratitis. Invest Ophthalmol Vis Sci 44:5228–5234
102. Whiting D, Hsieh G, Yun JJ, Banerji A, Yao W, Fishbein MC, Belperio J, Strieter RM, Bonavida B, Ardehali A (2004) Chemokine monokine induced by IFN-γ/CXC chemokine ligand 9 stimulates T lymphocyte proliferation and effector cytokine production. J Immunol 172:7417–7424
103. Wickham S, Carr DJJ (2004) Molecular mimicry versus bystander activation: herpetic stromal keratitis. Autoimmunity 37:393–397
104. Yan X T, M Tumpey T, L Kunkel S, Oakes JE, Lausch RN (1998) Role of MIP-2 in neutrophil migration and tissue injury in the herpes simplex virus-1-infected cornea. Invest Ophthalmol Vis Sci 39:1854–1862
105. Zeng X, Moore TA, Newstead MW, Deng JC, Lukacs NW, J Standiford T (2005) IP-10 mediates selective mononuclear cell accumulation and activation in response to intrapulmonary transgenic expression during adenovirus-induced pulmonary inflammation. J Interferon Cytokine Res 25:103–112
106. Zheng M, Klinman DM, Gierynska M, Rouse BT (2002) DNA containing CpG motifs induces angiogenesis. Proc Natl Acad Sci USA 99:8944–8949

Influence of Proinflammatory Cytokines and Chemokines on the Neuropathogenesis of Oncornavirus and Immunosuppressive Lentivirus Infections

K. E. Peterson[1] (✉) · B. Chesebro[2]

[1] Dept. of Pathobiological Sciences, School of Veterinary Medicine, Louisiana State University, Baton Rouge, LA 70803, USA
kpeterson@vetmed.lsu.edu

[2] Laboratory of Persistent Viral Diseases, Rocky Mountain Laboratories, NIAID, Hamilton, MT 59840, USA

1	Retrovirus Infections of the CNS	69
1.1	Historical Perspective	69
1.2	Diversity of Retrovirus-Induced Neurological Diseases	69
1.3	Diversity of Retrovirus-Induced Pathogenic Mechanisms	71
2	Fr98 Polytropic Retrovirus Model of Neuropathogenesis	72
2.1	Use of a Mouse Model to Study Retroviral Neuropathogenesis	72
2.2	FMCF98 and Fr98 Polytropic Murine Leukemia Viruses	72
2.3	Mapping of Neurovirulence Determinants in the Fr98 Genome	74
2.4	Contribution of Virus Burden to Pathogenesis	75
3	Cytokines and Chemokines in Fr98-Induced Neuropathogenesis	75
3.1	Analysis of Cytokine and Chemokine Gene Expression	75
3.2	Kinetics of Gene Expression	77
3.3	Studies with Knockout Mice	78
4	Cytokines and Chemokines in Immunosuppressive Lentivirus Pathogenesis	79
4.1	Correlation Between Gene Expression and Neurological Disease	79
4.2	Effect of HIV Proteins on Cytokine and Chemokine Induction	80
5	Potential Effects of Chemokines During Retrovirus Infection of the Brain	80
5.1	Activation and Recruitment of Microglia and Macrophages	80
5.2	Lymphocyte Recruitment	81
5.3	Neuronal Apoptosis	82
5.4	Direct Stimulation of Neurons	83
5.5	Alteration or Inhibition of Neuroprogenitor Stem Cell Migration	83
5.6	Astrocyte Activation and Support Functions	84
5.7	Retrovirus Entry and Spread in the CNS	85
5.8	Retroviral Protein Stimulation of Chemokine Receptors	85

| 6 | Conclusions | 86 |

References 87

Abstract Retroviral infection of the CNS can lead to severe debilitating neurological diseases in humans and other animals. Four general types of pathogenic effects with various retroviruses have been observed including: hemorrhage (TR1.3), spongiform encephalopathy (CasBrE, FrCasE, PVC211, NT40, Mol-ts1), demyelination with inflammatory lesions (HTLV-1, visna, CAEV), and encephalopathy with gliosis and proinflammatory chemokines and cytokines, usually with microglial giant cells and nodules [human immunodeficiency virus (HIV), feline immunodeficiency virus (FIV), simian immunodeficiency virus (SIV), Fr98]. This review focuses on this fourth group of retroviruses. In this latter group, proinflammatory cytokine and chemokine upregulation accompanies the disease process, and may influence pathogenesis by direct effects on resident CNS cells. The review first discusses the Fr98 murine polytropic virus system with particular reference to the roles of cytokines and chemokines in the pathogenic process. The Fr98 data are then compared and contrasted to the cytokine and chemokine data in the lentivirus systems, HIV, SIV, and FIV. Finally, various mechanisms are presented by which tumor necrosis factor (TNF) and several chemokines may alter the pathogenesis of retrovirus infection of the CNS.

Abbreviations

CAEV	Caprine arthritis encephalitis virus
CNS	Central nervous system
EIAV	Equine infectious anemia virus
GFAP	Glial fibrillary acidic protein
FIV	Feline immunodeficiency virus
FIV-E	FIV encephalitis
HAD	HIV-associated dementia
HIV	Human immunodeficiency virus
HTLV	Human T cell leukemia virus
IP	Intraperitoneal
LPS	Lipopolysaccharide
Mol-ts1	Moloney Ts1
NPSC	Neuroprogenitor stem cells
SIV	Simian immunodeficiency virus
SIV-E	SIV encephalitis

1
Retrovirus Infections of the CNS

1.1
Historical Perspective

In the initial years of the study of retroviruses the main emphasis was on the potential of these agents to induce neoplastic transformation of various tissues, especially muscle cells, fibroblasts, mammary glands, and bone marrow-derived hematopoietic cells. Subsequently non-neoplastic pathogenic effects of retroviruses were described, including anemia, arthritis, glomerulonephritis, immunodeficiencies, osteopetrosis, and neurological disorders. The studies of visna virus infection in sheep by Sigurdsson and colleagues in the 1950s demonstrated a slow CNS disease lasting several years (Sigurdsson et al. 1957, 1960). This long time course led ultimately to the name "lentiviruses" for the subgroup—including visna—of retroviruses with complex genomes. In the 1970s, Gardner and colleagues described a murine retrovirus from the oncornavirus subgroup (with simple genomes) which induced a slow neurological disease (Gardner et al. 1973). Since that time a large variety of other retroviruses from both subfamilies capable of inducing neurological disease in a variety of species including humans have been described (Table 1).

1.2
Diversity of Retrovirus-Induced Neurological Diseases

Retroviruses can cause several different types of neurological disease. Based on pathology and pathogenic effects, these can be divided into four groups (Table 1). These include: hemorrhage (TR1.3) (Park et al. 1993, 1994); spongiform encephalopathy (CasBrE, FrCasE, PVC211, NT40, Moloney-ts1) (Czub et al. 1995; Gardner 1988; Hoffman et al. 1992; Kai and Furuta 1984; Wong et al. 1985); demyelination with inflammatory lesions (HTLV-1, visna, CAEV) (Araujo and Hall 2004; Haase 1986; Jacobson 2002; Oaks et al. 2004); and encephalopathy associated with microgliosis, astrogliosis usually with microglial nodules, and giant cells and variable mononuclear cell infiltrates [human immunodeficiency virus (HIV), feline immunodeficiency virus (FIV), simian immunodeficiency virus (SIV), Fr98] (Glass et al. 1993, 1995; Kolson et al. 1998; Lackner et al. 1991; Portis et al. 1995; Robertson et al. 1997). Some viruses, such as SIV, appear to be able to induce more than one type of pathogenic process, depending on the viral strain used and/or the extent of immunosuppression (Lackner et al. 1991). In most models, infection of neurons is not observed and the mechanism of neuronal dysfunction is assumed to be indirect (Patrick et al. 2002; Portis 2001). In some systems, infection of

Table 1 Diversity of central nervous system pathological processes induced by retroviruses

Pathogenic effects	Virus	Species
Hemorrhage	TR1.3	Mouse
Spongiform encephalopathy	CasBrE	Mouse
	FrCasE	Mouse
	Mol-ts1	Mouse
	NT40	Rat
	PVC211	Rat
	TR1.3[a]	Mouse
Demyelination with extensive mononuclear cell infiltrates	CAEV	Goat
	EIAV[b]	Horse
	HERV[c]	Human
	HTLV-1	Human
	HTLV-2[d]	Human
	Visna	Sheep
Encephalopathy, gliosis, and upregulated proinflammatory cytokines and chemokines, with variable mononuclear cell infiltrates[e]	FIV	Cat
	Fr98	Mouse
	HIV	Human
	SIV	Monkey

[a] TR1.3 has been reported to induce both hemorrhage and spongiform encephalopathy (Murphy et al. 2004)
[b] Equine infectious anemia virus (EIAV) sporadically induces a brain inflammatory disease but demyelination was not noted (Oaks et al. 2004)
[c] HERVs, human endogenous retroviruses, may be involved in multiple sclerosis (Christensen 2005)
[d] HTLV-2 is believed to be associated with some rare cases of demyelinating encephalitis (Araujo and Hall 2004)
[e] The extent of mononuclear cell infiltration in the lentiviral models (HIV, SIV, FIV) can vary considerably from prominent to minimal (Anthony et al. 2005; Gardner and Dandekar 1995; Kolson et al. 1998; Lackner et al. 1991). In the Fr98 neonatal mouse model mononuclear infiltration is minimal (Peterson et al. 2001; Robertson et al. 1997)

neurons has been noted, but this does not appear to account for the disease, because the infected cells are not present in the damaged areas (Lynch et al. 1991). Despite the diverse pathology, most retroviruses infect the same major target cells of microglia and macrophages in the brain (Patrick et al. 2002; Portis 2001). Brain capillary endothelial cells are often extensively infected in many murine models and may be in some primate systems (SIV). To a lesser extent, infection of astrocytes (Liu et al. 2004) and oligodendrocytes (Robertson et al. 1997) has also been observed with some retroviruses, but these types of infected cells may nevertheless play important roles in the pathogenesis.

1.3
Diversity of Retrovirus-Induced Pathogenic Mechanisms

Mechanisms of pathogenesis are not well understood in most of these retroviral systems. The simplest model appears to be the TR1.3 murine retrovirus, where infection of brain capillary endothelial cells leads to cell fusion and damaged and leaky blood vessels (Park et al. 1993, 1994). However, more recent data indicate that TR1.3 can also induce spongiform encephalopathy (Murphy et al. 2004). In some rodent spongiform encephalopathy models, such as PVC211, there is evidence that endothelial cell infection is important to pathogenesis probably by facilitating viral entry into the CNS (Hoffman et al. 1992; Kai and Furuta 1984). In other rodent spongiform encephalopathy models, such as FrCasE, Cas-Br-E, and Moloney ts1, there is growing evidence that viral envelope protein aggregation may lead to an endoplasmic reticulum stress response, which may in turn damage certain glial cells (Dimcheff et al. 2003, 2004; Kim et al. 2004a; Liu et al. 2004). However, the explanation for the very restricted spatial distribution of lesions in the face of widespread virus infection remains unclear. The demyelinating inflammatory viruses all appear to induce a very strong host inflammatory response involving lymphocytes and macrophages, and the cytokines and chemokines produced by infiltrating cells are believed to be important in demyelination and neuronal damage (Araujo and Hall 2004; Haase 1986; Jacobson 2002).

The immunodeficiency inducing lentiviruses, HIV, SIV, and FIV, as well as Fr98, a polytropic murine retrovirus, all induce a severe clinical CNS disease with minimal morphological neuronal damage and pathology. Multiple histopathological changes have been associated with HIV-associated dementia (HAD), including microglia nodules, astrogliosis, microgliosis, neuronal apoptosis, myelin pallor, and multinucleated giant cell formation (Anthony et al. 2005; Glass et al. 1995; Kolson et al. 1998). Many of these alterations have also been seen in animal models (Johnston et al. 2002; Lackner et al. 1991; Portis et al. 1995; Power et al. 2004; Robertson et al. 1997; Williams et al. 2001). The main pathological change-associated clinical neurological disease is the increased presence of activated macrophages and microglia in the brain (Anthony et al. 2005; Glass et al. 1995; Portis et al. 1995; Robertson et al. 1997; Williams et al. 2001). Virus infection does not generally induce extensive infiltration of inflammatory cells from outside the CNS (Anthony et al. 2005; Glass et al. 1995; Power and Johnson 1995, 2001; Robertson et al. 1997); however, there is evidence for a role for proinflammatory cytokines and chemokines in the pathogenesis of these viruses. The low level of inflammatory infiltrates in all of these models is likely related to the presence of severe immunosuppression induced by the virus (HIV, SIV, FIV) or the neonatal state of the host (Fr98 infection). This review will focus on the role of proinflammatory cytokines and chemokines in the neuropathogenesis of this group of retroviruses with emphasis on the Fr98 mouse model and the use of knockout mice to study the contribution of cytokines and chemokines to retroviral pathogenesis.

2
Fr98 Polytropic Retrovirus Model of Neuropathogenesis

2.1
Use of a Mouse Model to Study Retroviral Neuropathogenesis

In human patients, it is difficult to distinguish cause versus effect in correlative studies of gene upregulation. Other animal models of retrovirus infection, including SIV infection of macaques and FIV infection of felines have this same limitation. Mouse models of retrovirus infection offer the unique advantage over other retrovirus systems in the ability to use knockout and transgenic animals to definitively determine whether specific proteins are necessary for disease development. The mouse model of polytropic retrovirus infection also allows the comparison between non-neurovirulent and neurovirulent retrovirus infections (Peterson et al. 2001, 2004b; Robertson et al. 1997). This permits the determination of whether a host response is specific to pathogenesis or is a general response to retrovirus infection. Additionally, the availability of inbred mouse strains, the short gestation period of mice, and the short incubation time of neurological disease induction in mice compared to humans or non-human primates allows for the kinetic and statistical analysis of the host response genes.

2.2
FMCF98 and Fr98 Polytropic Murine Leukemia Viruses

In 1990, during studies of retrovirus-induced leukemia using Friend murine leukemia virus (MuLV) inoculation of neonatal mice, a novel retrovirus was isolated which appeared to cause both a neurological disease and leukemia (Buller et al. 1990). After biological and molecular cloning, the causative virus, FMCF98, was found to have a polytropic host range, as it was capable of infecting cell lines from mice as well as from a variety of other species, and it caused the typical mink cell foci (MCF) associated with other polytropic mouse retroviruses (Portis et al. 1995). After intraperitoneal (IP) infection of susceptible mouse strains the infection expanded first in hematopoietic cells of bone marrow and spleen and then progressed via blood to the brain.

Table 2 Polytropic retroviruses

Virus	Viral genome	CNS disease	Virus load	Upregulation of cytokines and chemokines
FMCF98		Yes (6–24 weeks)	++	Not tested
FB29		No	+++++	No
Fr98		Yes (2–3 weeks)	+++	High[a]
Fr54		No	++	No
SE		Yes (3–8 weeks)	+++	High[a]
BE		Yes (3–8 weeks)	+++	High[a]
EC		Yes (3–8 weeks)	++	Low[b]

[a] Genes upregulated: $Tnf\alpha$, $Tnf\beta$, $IL\text{-}1\alpha$, $Ccl2$, $Ccl3$, $Ccl4$, $Ccl5$, $Cxcl10$
[b] Expression of cytokine and chemokine mRNA not statistically different as compared to mock-infected controls in whole brain; however, some cytokines, such as TNF-α, are upregulated in the middle region of the brain including the hippocampus, thalamus, and hypothalamus

The neurological disease consisted of ataxia, hind limb weakness, tremors, seizures, and death occurred in nearly 80% of mice by 6 months. In genetic studies, IRW mice were highly susceptible and C57BL/10 were highly resistant and two uncharacterized host genes appeared to account for most of this resistance (Buller et al. 1990). Because studies of a disease taking 6–8 months were difficult, a virus with a more rapid phenotype was derived by cloning the envelope gene of FMCF98 into the backbone of a rapidly replicating retrovirus, FB29 (Table 2) (Portis et al. 1995). By 20–30 days postinfection with this virus, Fr98, mice had the same neurological symptoms and pathology as produced by FMCF98. Within the brain, endothelial cells and microglia were the main target cells of Fr98, although rare infection of oligodendrocytes was also detected (Robertson et al. 1997). The brain pathology consisted of prominent reactive astrogliosis and widespread white matter microglial infection with microgliosis and occasional microglial giant cells and nodules, and minimal vacuolation (Portis et al. 1995). Neuronal cell death was not a prominent feature (Portis et al. 1995).

2.3
Mapping of Neurovirulence Determinants in the Fr98 Genome

Since neurological disease was not induced by most murine retroviruses, it was of interest to determine which regions of the Fr98 genome were important for this brain disease. Fr98 was compared to Fr54, a non-neurovirulent chimeric polytropic retrovirus with a similar structure (Hasenkrug et al. 1996). Fr54 contained the envelope *(env)* gene of FMCF54 inserted into FB29, and differed from Fr98 by several amino acid residues in the polymerase *(pol)* and *env* genes. Fr54 was able to infect the same cell types in the brain as Fr98; however, no neurological symptoms were observed. The level of Fr54 virus infection was slightly lower than that of Fr98, but there was no clear difference in the neuropathology (Hasenkrug et al. 1996; Robertson et al. 1997). Thus the pathology appeared to be due to retroviral infection, independent of the disease induction, suggesting perhaps that the disease symptoms and death were due to biochemical abnormalities not represented by obvious morphological changes.

In order to determine which regions of the Fr98 genome were responsible for induction of the neurological disease, several chimeric recombinant viruses using sequences of either Fr98 or Fr54 were studied (Hasenkrug et al. 1996; Peterson et al. 2004b). These data indicated that there were two non-overlapping regions of the Fr98 genome which influenced neurovirulence, one from *SphI* to *EcoRI* (SE), and the other from *EcoRI* to *ClaI* (EC) (Table 2). Both these chimeras induced disease slower than Fr98, suggesting that they acted by different but complementary mechanisms. The EC region contained only *env* sequences, whereas the SE region contained both *pol* and *env* sequences. However, only *env* sequences were involved in neurovirulence because a chimera with Fr98 sequences from *BbsI* to *EcoRI* (BE), containing only *env*, was similar in virulence to SE (Peterson et al. 2004b) (Table 2). The BE region contains 11 *env* amino acid differences between Fr98 and Fr54, and current studies are investigating which residues are most important to disease induction (K. Peterson and B. Chesebro, in preparation). The EC region contained 17 *env* amino acid differences, and mutagenesis studies identified changes at two positions (residues 195 and 198) as being important for disease induction (Poulsen et al. 1998).

The mechanisms of disease induced by these two *env* regions are still unclear; however, some clues were provided by previous studies. Earlier data indicated that the SE/BE region appeared to influence the brain viral load and the kinetics of replication, and for these chimeras a high viral load was required for disease. In contrast, the EC region induced disease at a lower viral load, and thus appeared to generate neurotoxicity which did not require high virus replication (Poulsen et al. 1998).

2.4
Contribution of Virus Burden to Pathogenesis

A role for higher viral load influencing disease was also shown in studies using direct brain infection by intraventricular inoculation of virus-infected neural stem cells (Poulsen et al. 1999). In these experiments virus infection of brain endothelial cells was minimal, whereas infection of microglial cells was greatly increased for all viruses tested. Interestingly, with this method even the avirulent virus Fr54 was capable of inducing neurological disease, albeit considerably more slowly than Fr98. These data indicated that all the polytropic retroviruses studied had potential to induce neurological disease if expressed in the brain at a high enough level. Perhaps the role of the SE/BE *env* region is to elevate viral replication to these high levels even when the standard route of IP infection is used. In contrast, since the EC chimera induced disease even at lower viral loads, it would appear that the critical Fr98 amino acids at positions 195 and 198 in this chimera have a higher potential for disease induction than the comparable Fr54 residues.

3
Cytokines and Chemokines in Fr98-Induced Neuropathogenesis

3.1
Analysis of Cytokine and Chemokine Gene Expression

Fr98-induced neurological disease is not associated with the widespread spongiform degeneration, intracerebral hemorrhaging, or extensive leukocyte infiltration associated with other neurovirulent murine retroviruses. Instead, the primary pathology associated with Fr98 infection is gliosis with increased presence of activated microglia, macrophages, and astrocytes in the brain (Portis et al. 1995; Robertson et al. 1997). As the pathology between Fr54 and Fr98 infection is similar (Portis et al. 1995; Robertson et al. 1997), the pathogenic mechanism by which Fr98 induces disease does not appear to cause distinctive morphological alterations. Possibly this pathogenesis acts at a molecular level through the regulation of gene expression. Molecular analysis of gene expression by RNAse protection assay confirmed the lack of lymphocytic infiltration in the brain with no detectable increase in messenger (m)RNA for T cell- or B cell-specific genes or T cell-associated cytokines or cytokine receptors in brain tissue from Fr98-infected mice compared to mock-, Fr54-, or FB29-infected mice (Peterson et al. 2001). Additionally, no significant changes in gene expression were detected in the apoptosis-related genes, *Fas, Fasl, Fadd, Tradd, Bax, Bcl-X, Bcl-2* ,and *Bcl-W*. Fr98 pathogenesis was associated with a heightened proinflammatory response with increased mRNA expression of TNF(TNFSF1A,TNFα), TNFSF1B(TNFβ, lymphotoxin A), IL1β, CCL2(MCP-1), CCL3(MIP-1α), CCL4(MIP-1β), CCL5(RANTES), CXCL1(MIP-2), and CXCL10(IP-10) in the brain tissue of Fr98-infected mice (Peterson et al. 2001). Induction of cytokines and chemokines correlated with neurovirulence, not virus presence, as no significant mRNA upregulation of these genes was observed in FB29- or Fr54-infected mice. Protein levels of TNF(TNFα), CCL2(MCP-1), CCL3(MIP-1α), CCL4(MIP-1β), and CCL5(RANTES) were also increased in brain tissue from Fr98-infected mice (Fig. 1), indicating a correlation between the upregulation of cytokine and chemokine mRNA and protein expression. By in situ hybridization analysis, CCL2(MCP-1) and CXCL10(IP-10) mRNA was expressed by astrocytes, while CCL3(MIP-1α), CCL4(MIP-1β), and CCL5(RANTES) mRNA was expressed by uninfected cells, possibly microglia or macrophages (Peterson et al. 2004a; K. Peterson and B. Chesebro, unpublished observations).

Comparison of proinflammatory cytokine and chemokine expression following infection of the chimeric polytropic retroviruses indicated a corre-

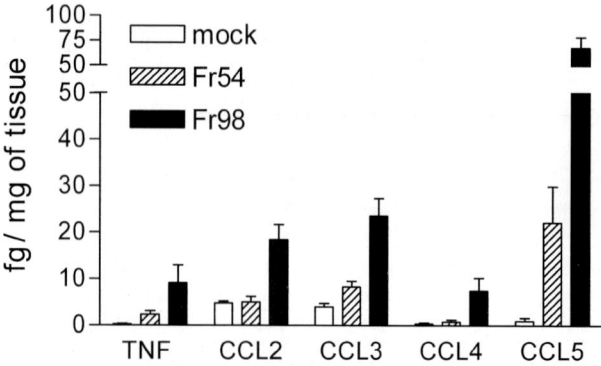

Fig. 1 Increased protein expression of TNF and chemokines in Fr98-infected mice. Enzyme-linked immunosorbent assay (ELISA) kits specific for the appropriate murine protein were purchased from R&D Systems (Minneapolis, MN). Brain tissue from Fr98-, Fr54-, or mock-infected mice were removed at 14 days postinfection, snap frozen in liquid nitrogen, and stored at −80°C until use. The samples were homogenized in 0.1 M Tris pH 7.4, 0.15 M NaCl, 0.5% NP40 with complete protease inhibitor (Roche Applied Science, Indianapolis, IN) to a final concentration of 30% w/v. Samples were incubated overnight at 4°C, and 50 µl per sample was added to duplicate wells for each protein-specific ELISA. Data are presented as femtograms of the protein of interest per milligram of brain tissue and are the mean +/− standard error of 4–8 samples per group. A significant increase ($p<0.05$) in protein levels of brain tissue from Fr98-infected mice was observed for all proteins analyzed

lation between the SE/BE neurovirulent determinant of the Fr98 envelope and the induction of cytokine and chemokine mRNA expression (Peterson et al. 2001). Increased cytokine and chemokine expression was observed in the brain tissue of SE and BE-infected mice (Peterson et al. 2001, 2004b). In contrast, cytokine expression in EC-infected mice was more restricted, with localized upregulation of tumor necrosis factor (TNF) in the middle (hippocampus, midbrain, and thalamus) region of the brain (Peterson et al. 2001, 2004b). As Fr98, SE and BE replicate in the brain at a two- to threefold higher level than EC or Fr54 (Table 2) (Hasenkrug et al. 1996; Peterson et al. 2004b; Robertson et al. 1997), the upregulation of cytokine and chemokine expression may be due to the increased viral burden associated with these viruses. Alternatively, specific envelope determinants may be necessary for the induction of these proinflammatory factors.

3.2
Kinetics of Gene Expression

The correlation between increased proinflammatory cytokines and chemokines and retrovirus-induced neuropathogenesis suggests that these proinflammatory factors may induce pathogenesis or be induced as a result of pathogenic insult. One way to dissect the cause versus effect relationship of these events is the analysis of the timing of upregulation of cytokines and chemokines relative to disease onset. Kinetic analysis of gene expression is difficult in HIV, SIV, and FIV studies due to limitations in tissue sampling as well as the variation in disease progression and the incidence of disease. However, in the Fr98 mouse model, after infection with high virus doses, 100% of the animals develop neurological disease within 14 to 16 days postinfection (Peterson et al. 2001; Poulsen et al. 1999). An increase in mRNA expression of TNF, CCL2(MCP-1), CCL3(MIP-1α), CCL4(MIP-1β), CCL5(RANTES), CXCL1(MIP-2), and CXCL10(IP-10) was detected in preclinical mice, 3–4 days prior to the neurological disease, suggesting that these cytokines and chemokines might contribute to disease induction (Peterson et al. 2001). In contrast, increased expression of TNFSF1B(TNFβ, lymphotoxin A) and interleukin (IL)-1α mRNA was only consistently found in Fr98-infected mice with clinical disease, suggesting that these cytokines may be a response to disease rather than a cause of pathogenesis. Interestingly, mRNA expression of two additional chemokines, CCL7(MCP-3) and CCL12(MCP-5), was upregulated 3 to 4 days prior to clinical disease development, but returned to basal levels at the time of clinical disease (Peterson et al. 2004a). Similarly, CCL12(MCP-5)-positive cells were found in brain tissue of preclinical mice, but were difficult to detect in mice with clinical disease. Although

CCL7(MCP-3) and CCL12(MCP-5) are not upregulated at the time of disease, they could contribute to the early stages of disease development prior to the onset of clinical disease.

3.3
Studies with Knockout Mice

Knockout mouse and antibody blocking studies indicated a role for specific cytokines and chemokines in Fr98-mediated pathogenesis in the brain. Mice deficient in CCR2, the primary ligand for CCL2(MCP-1) and CCL12(MCP-5), had reduced incidence and kinetics of neurological disease following Fr98 infection, indicating that CCR2 stimulation was contributing to pathogenesis (Peterson et al. 2004a). Antibody blocking studies indicated that the CCR2 ligand CCL2(MCP-1), but not ligands CCL7(MCP-3) or CCL12(MCP-5), contributed to Fr98-induced disease. Thus, CCL2(MCP-1) stimulation of CCR2 appears to be a mechanism of Fr98-mediated neuropathogenesis. In contrast, CCR5 was not necessary for Fr98 pathogenesis as no decrease in neurovirulence was observed in CCR5-deficient mice, despite increased mRNA and protein expression of the CCR5 ligands CCL3(MIP-1α), CCL4(MIP-1β), and CCL5(RANTES) (Peterson et al. 2001, 2004a; Fig. 1).

In TNF-deficient mice, the rate of Fr98-induced disease progression was significantly delayed, demonstrating that TNF contributed to neuropathogenesis (Peterson et al. 2004b). Interestingly, the role of TNF in pathogenesis varied with different chimeric polytropic retroviruses. For example, the chimeric virus BE induced high levels of TNF mRNA in the brain, whereas the chimeric virus EC induced only localized production of TNF mRNA in the middle (midbrain, hippocampus, and thalamus) region of the brain. This correlation suggested that TNF deficiency might inhibit BE-induced disease and not EC-induced disease. However, paradoxically, the opposite was observed. TNF deficiency significantly inhibited EC-induced clinical disease, but had no detectable effect on BE-induced disease (Peterson et al. 2004b). This result demonstrated the danger of drawing conclusions strictly from correlative data.

EC-induced upregulation of the microglia and macrophage marker F4/80 was not observed in TNF-deficient mice, suggesting that TNF may contribute to disease by the activation or recruitment of microglia or macrophages (Peterson et al. 2004b). In contrast, TNF was not necessary for retrovirus-induced activation of astrocytes as measured by expression of glial fibrillary acidic protein (GFAP) mRNA. Further studies analyzing the responses of retrovirus infection in knockout mice should provide valuable information in regards to how cytokines and chemokines contribute to neuropathogenesis.

Increased TNF mRNA expression has also been associated with the spongiform degeneration and neurological disease induced by the FrCasE and Mol-ts1 murine retrovirus infections (Askovic et al. 2001; Choe et al. 1998; Peterson et al. 2004b). However, deficiencies in TNF or TNFR1 did not alter the pathogenesis of disease induced by FrCasE and Mol-ts1, respectively (Jolicoeur et al. 2003; Peterson et al. 2004b).

4
Cytokines and Chemokines in Immunosuppressive Lentivirus Pathogenesis

4.1
Correlation Between Gene Expression and Neurological Disease

Similar to the upregulation of cytokines and chemokines in the Fr98 model, several studies have demonstrated expression of proinflammatory cytokines and chemokines in HAD. Increased mRNA or protein expression of CCL2(MCP-1), CCL3(MIP-1α), CCL4(MIP-1β), CCL5(RANTES), CXCL10(IP-10), TNF(TNF α), interferon (IFN)-γ, and IL-1 have been observed in brain tissue or cerebrospinal fluid of HIV-infected patients with dementia (Conant et al. 1998; Kolb et al. 1999; McManus et al. 2000; Schmidtmayerova et al. 1996; Tyor et al. 1992; Vago et al. 2001). A strong correlation was also observed between TNF mRNA expression and clinical signs of dementia (Glass et al. 1993), although, based on studies using TNF knockout mice in the Fr98 system, gene expression of TNF does not always correlate with a role of TNF in neuropathogenesis. The source of CCL2(MCP-1) expression in HAD patients was astrocytes (Conant et al. 1998), while CCL5(RANTES) was expressed by lymphocytes and uninfected microglia/macrophages (Vago et al. 2001) and TNF, IFN-γ, and IL-1 were produced by perivascular macrophages and endothelia (Tyor et al. 1992).

Increased cytokine and chemokine mRNA and protein expression also correlated with encephalitis induced by SIV or FIV infection. Increased cerebrospinal fluid levels of CCL2(MCP-1) was a strong indicator of SIV-induced encephalitis (Zink et al. 2001). Additionally, increased mRNA and/or protein expression of CCL3(MIP-1α), CCL4(MIP-1β), CCL5(RANTES), CCL7(MCP-3), CXCL10(IP-10), IL-1β, IL-4, IL-6, IFN-γ, and TNF have been associated with encephalitis in the SIV model (Lane et al. 1996; Orandle et al. 2002; Sasseville et al. 1996; Sopper et al. 1996; Sui et al. 2003), with TNF expression by macrophages in perivascular lesions (Orandle et al. 2002). Similarly, increased expression of TNF mRNA by microglia and astrocytes appears to be involved in the early stages of FIV-induced encephalitis in cats (Poli et al. 1999).

4.2
Effect of HIV Proteins on Cytokine and Chemokine Induction

In the Fr98 model, particular sequences in the viral envelope protein influenced the production of cytokines and chemokines, possibly through the regulation of virus levels in the brain (Peterson et al. 2001). In the SCID-HIVE model, increased expression of both CCL2(MCP-1) and CCL3(MIP-1α) was associated with HIV-infected monocytes in the brain (Persidsky et al. 1999). Similar induction of cytokines and chemokines such as CCL2(MCP-1), CXCL10(IP-10), CXCL9(MIG), and IL-1β were observed in mouse brain tissue following inoculation with HIV-1 provirus or a chimeric HIV virus with an ecotropic MuLV envelope protein (Potash et al. 2005; Wang et al. 2003). Both the Tat and Env protein of HIV appeared to contribute to the upregulation of cytokines and chemokines. HIV Tat stimulation of in vitro cultures of glial cell cultures induced the expression of several chemokines including CCL2(MCP-1) and CCL3(MIP-1α) (McManus et al. 2000), while stimulation of astrocytes with HIV gp120 induced CXCL10(IP-10) expression (Asensio et al. 2001). A similar induction of CXCL10(IP-10) as well as CCL2(MCP-1) was observed in mice with transgenic expression of gp120 under the GFAP promoter (Asensio et al. 2001). Interestingly, no clinical signs of neurological disease were reported in these in vivo models, indicating that increased production of chemokines in the brain at the levels achieved in these experiments was not sufficient for the induction of neurological disease.

5
Potential Effects of Chemokines During Retrovirus Infection of the Brain

Polymorphism studies have suggested that certain alleles of TNF and CCL2(MCP-1) correlate with increased risk of the development of dementia in HIV-infected patients (Gonzalez et al. 2002; Quasney et al. 2001). Studies with the Fr98 mouse model also demonstrated that CCL2(MCP-1), its primary receptor, CCR2, and TNF contributed to retroviral pathogenesis in the brain (Peterson et al. 2004a, b). Comparison of wildtype and knockout mice in the Fr98 pathogenesis model as well as in vitro and in vivo studies with HIV, SIV, and FIV have indicated several mechanisms by which these proteins may contribute to pathogenesis.

5.1
Activation and Recruitment of Microglia and Macrophages

The lack of neurological disease in TNF-deficient mice following EC retrovirus infection was associated with a lack of increased expression of the microglia and macrophage marker F4/80 (Peterson et al. 2004b). Thus, TNF may have an important role in the activation and/or recruitment of brain microglia and macrophages. Autopsy findings from HAD patients indicated a strong correlation between increased staining for activated macrophages and microglial cells in the brain and the severity of dementia (Glass et al. 1995). Similarly, an increase in activated macrophages and/or microglia has also been associated with encephalitis following SIV or FIV infection (Georgsson 1994; Lackner et al. 1991; Williams and Hickey 2002). Blood–brain barrier (BBB) permeability and tight junction disruption have been noted in cases of HIV and SIV infections (Boven et al. 2000; Luabeya et al. 2000), indicating that infected and uninfected peripheral macrophages may migrate to the brain and contribute to retroviral pathogenesis. In the SCID-HIVE mouse model, HIV-infected cells in the CNS were surrounded by murine macrophages, suggesting the migration of either peripheral or brain macrophages to the site of virus in the brain (Nukuna et al. 2004). TNF expression has been demonstrated to break down the BBB as well as induce microglia and macrophage activation and macrophage migration in vitro (Glabinski et al. 1998; Hurwitz et al. 1994).

Chemokines may play an important role in the migration of peripherally activated macrophages across the BBB. The term chemokine was coined to describe a family of chemoattractant cytokines that were involved in the recruitment and tissue extravasation of leukocytes during inflammation. The chemokine CCL2(MCP-1) induced monocyte migration across an endothelial cell/astrocyte co-culture model of the BBB (Eugenin and Berman 2003). Expression of CCR2, the primary receptor for CCL2(MCP-1), by macrophages was required for CCL2(MCP-1)-induced macrophage migration across a brain endothelial layer (Dzenko et al. 2005). Interestingly, CCR2 expression was also required on the brain microvessels, as neither CCR2$^+$ nor CCR2$^-$ macrophages could migrate across CCR2$^-$ brain endothelial cells in response CCL2(MCP-1) stimulation (Dzenko et al. 2005). It is possible that CCL2(MCP-1) and TNF contribute to retroviral pathogenesis by the same mechanism, with both cytokines involved in the activation and/or migration of microglia and macrophages in the brain.

5.2
Lymphocyte Recruitment

Expression of cytokines and chemokines may also recruit CD3 lymphocytes to the brain (Dufour et al. 2002; Moser et al. 2004; Ransohoff 2002; Ransohoff and Tani 1998). Although a detectable increase in CD8$^+$CD3$^+$ lymphocytic infiltration is not observed in the Fr98 model, increased numbers of CD8$^+$ lymphocytes in the CNS have been reported with both HIV-1 and SIV infections (Kim et al. 2004b; Miller et al. 2004; Petito et al. 2003). However, persistent depletion of CD8$^+$ lymphocytes correlated with increased encephalitis in brains of SIV-infected macaques (Williams et al. 2001; Williams and Hickey 2002). Thus, rather than contributing to retroviral pathogenesis, CD8$^+$ T cells may suppress the recruitment and trafficking of infected macrophages in the CNS, delaying the development of neurological symptoms.

5.3
Neuronal Apoptosis

Apoptotic neurons and neuronal dropout have been observed in brain tissue of HAD patients and animal models of retroviral neuropathogenesis, although there does not appear to be a direct correlation with the amount of neuronal apoptosis and clinical neurological disease (Adle-Biassette et al. 1999; Kolson et al. 1998). In contrast, no detectable increase in neuronal apoptosis was associated with Fr98 infection or disease (Peterson et al. 2004b; Portis et al. 1995), but lack of apoptosis might be due to the short disease course in this model. This result suggests that the severe clinical symptoms observed by Fr98 infection are not the result of neuronal death, but instead more likely represent neuronal dysfunction. In slower disease models, apoptosis may be the end result of neuronal damage induced by cytokines and chemokines, but this interpretation is not conclusive because these proinflammatory molecules can have opposing effects in different situations. For example, TNF has been directly implicated in inducing apoptosis through stimulation of TNFRI, but may be anti-apoptotic when stimulating through TNFRII (Saha and Pahan 2003). CCL2(MCP-1) inhibited neuronal apoptosis induced by either N-methyl-D-aspartate (NMDA) or HIV Tat in mixed glial cultures (Eugenin et al. 2003). Similar results were also observed by the addition of CCL5(RANTES), suggesting that the production of chemokines during retrovirus infection may provide protection from retrovirus-induced neuronal apoptosis and may, in some instances, decrease the pathogenesis of retrovirus infection. In vitro studies have shown that chemokines such as CCL5(RANTES), CXCL12(SDF1α), and CCL22(MDC) can provide support for the survival of neuronal cultures in the absence of glial feeder cells (Meucci et al. 1998).

Retrovirus proteins including HIV-1 Tat and gp120 can induce apoptosis when added to neurons in vitro (Catani et al. 2000; Meucci et al. 1998; Zhang et al. 2003). HIV gp120-induced neuronal apoptosis was blocked by anti-CXCR4 or anti-CCR5 antibodies, indicating that HIV gp120 neurotoxicity may be mediated by chemokine receptor signaling (Zhang et al. 2003). CCL3(MIP-1α), CCL4(MIP-1β), CCL5(RANTES), and CXCL12(SDF1α) inhibited gp120-induced apoptosis (Catani et al. 2000; Meucci et al. 1998), suggesting that the expression of these chemokines during retrovirus infection may block the neurotoxic effects of gp120. Thus, the ratio of chemokine expression to virus envelope production and the levels of cytokines or chemokines produced may regulate the amount of neuronal apoptosis associated with retrovirus infection.

5.4
Direct Stimulation of Neurons

Chemokines may also contribute to retrovirus neuropathogenesis through the direct stimulation of neuronal subsets in the brain. Embryonic and adult neurons have been reported to express a number of chemokine receptors including CCR1, CCR2, CCR5, CXCR3, and CXCR4 (Meucci et al. 1998; Tran et al. 2004; Tran and Miller 2003). Studies with hippocampal neurons demonstrated functional chemokine receptors as stimulation of neurons with CCL3(MIP-1α), CCL5(RANTES), CCL22(MDC), and CXCL12(SDF1α) induced calcium signaling (Meucci et al. 1998). Although CCL2(MCP-1) did not induce calcium signaling in hippocampal neurons (Meucci et al. 1998), studies with Purkinje neurons indicated that CCL2 could enhance calcium signaling following glutamate receptor activation (van Gassen et al. 2005). Patch-clamp experiments of cultured hypothalamic neurons indicated that chemokines such as CXCL12(SDF1α) might be directly involved in neuronal signaling (Guyon et al. 2005). Thus, the production of chemokines following retrovirus infection of the CNS may alter neuronal signaling patterns, leading to neurological disease.

5.5
Alteration or Inhibition of Neuroprogenitor Stem Cell Migration

Another mechanism by which CCL2(MCP-1)/CCR2 interactions may contribute to retroviral neuropathogenesis is through the alteration of neural progenitor stem cell (NPSC) migration in the brain or by effecting axonal growth and NPSC survival. This might be especially relevant in congenital HIV infection and also in the Fr98 mouse model, where mice are infected as neonates and the brain is still undergoing development. Abnormal brain development has not been reported in CCR1-, CCR2-, CCR3-, CCL2(MCP-1)-, or CXCL10(IP-10)-deficient mice, suggesting that these chemokines are not necessary for the normal migration of NPSC during development (Abbadie et al. 2003; Dufour et al. 2002; Humbles et al. 2002; Khan et al. 2001; Kuziel et al. 1997, 2003; Lu et al. 1998). However, CCL2(MCP-1) altered the migration of NPSC in vitro (Widera et al. 2004), suggesting that overexpression of chemokines may alter NPSC migration. Additionally, lipopolysaccharide

(LPS) was shown to inhibit NPSC migration patterns in vivo, possibly through the increased production of proinflammatory cytokines and chemokines in the brain (Monje et al. 2003). Chemokines have been shown to contribute to NPSC migration in vivo. Mice deficient in the chemokine receptor CXCR4, the receptor for the chemokine CXCL12(SDF1α), have deformed cerebellum development and lack neuronal migration from the external granular layer (Lu et al. 2002). The loss of CXCL12(SDF1α) also affects adult neurogenesis in the hippocampal dentate gyrus (Bagri et al. 2002). A decrease in migrating NPSC was detected in HIV-infected patients with dementia compared to those without, indicating that NPSC migration may influence disease (Krathwohl and Kaiser 2004). Alteration or suppression of NPSC migration could affect the development of the dentate gyrus and cerebellum and lead to the inhibition of memory and developmental skills associated with HIV infection in infants (Drapeau et al. 2003; Monje et al. 2003; Rola et al. 2004; Tran and Miller 2003).

5.6
Astrocyte Activation and Support Functions

Although most retroviruses do not productively infect astrocytes, reactive astrocytes as characterized by increased GFAP expression is commonly associated with neuropathogenesis induced by HIV, SIV, FIV, and Fr98, as well as other retroviruses (Kolson et al. 1998; Poli et al. 1997; Rausch et al. 1994; Robertson et al. 1997). Astrocytes are also the common source for CCL2(MCP-1) production during retrovirus infection and may contribute to pathogenesis by this mechanism (Conant et al. 1998; Peterson et al. 2004a; Zink et al. 2001). CXCL10(IP-10) production by retrovirus-stimulated astrocytes has also been detected (Asensio et al. 2001; Kutsch et al. 2000). Astrocytes express multiple functional chemokine receptors including CCR1, CCR2, CCR3, CCR5, CCR10, and CXCR4 (Andjelkovic et al. 2002; Croitoru-Lamoury et al. 2003; Dorf et al. 2000; Tanabe et al. 1997). Thus, the production of chemokines by astrocytes and other glial cells in the brain may affect the function of these cells.

Astrocytes play an important support function for neurons, by removing potentially neurotoxic glutamate from extracellular spaces and converting it to glutamine. Activated astrocytes express two glutamate receptors: SLC1A2 (solute carrier family 1–glial high-affinity glutamate transporter member 2, also known as GLT-1 or EAAT-2), which is found on astrocytes throughout the brain; and SLC1A3 (solute carrier family 1–glial high-affinity glutamate transporter member 3, also known as GLAST or EAAT-1), which can also be detected on neurons (Liberto et al. 2004). Trauma to cultured astrocytes results in increased mRNA and protein expression of both SLC1A2 and SLC1A3. Glutamate-ammonia ligase (GLUL, also known as glutamine synthase, GLNS), which converts glutamate to the non-neurotoxic glutamine, can also be upregulated in activated astrocytes. Altered expression of SLCA3 or other glutamate regulatory genes has been associated with neuropathogenesis, including SIV infection of the brain (Chretien et al. 2002, 2004; Guo et al. 2003; Li et al. 1997; Martin et al. 2000). Chemokine activation of astrocytes may affect the regulation of the glutamine synthesis and lead to the build-up of neurotoxic glutamate.

5.7
Retrovirus Entry and Spread in the CNS

In the Fr98 model, the lack of CCR2, CCR5, or TNF did not influence virus burden in the brain (Peterson et al. 2004a, b). However, Fr98 has not been reported to use chemokine receptors as coreceptors for virus entry. In contrast, HIV and SIV utilize the chemokine receptors CXCR4 and CCR5 as coreceptors for infection of T cells and macrophages, respectively (Alkhatib et al. 1996; Feng et al. 1996; Oberlin et al. 1996). In addition, other chemokine receptors including CCR2b, CCR3, and CCR8 have been shown to contribute to HIV or SIV infection and are often referred to as minor coreceptors (Gorry et al. 2001; Margulies et al. 2001). HIV patients with a CCR5 allele containing a 32-bp deletion had reduced incidence of HIV encephalitis (HIV-E), indicating that CCR5 is an important contributor to retrovirus infection of macrophages and/or microglia in vivo (van Rij et al. 1999). Chemokine expression in the brain during HIV-1 infection could impact virus infection of brain macrophages or microglia. CCL3(MIP-1α), CCL4(MIP-1β), and CCL5(RANTES) are ligands for CCR5 and are detected at increased levels in patients with HAD (Schmidtmayerova et al. 1996; Vago et al. 2001). The expression of these CCR5 ligands in the brain during HIV infection could block virus envelope binding of CCR5 molecules on macrophages and thus restrict the spread of HIV infection in the brain. Alternatively, stimulation of CCR5-positive macrophages by these ligands may induce increased expression of CCR5 on the cell surface, providing ample coreceptors for virus infection of brain macrophages.

5.8
Retroviral Protein Stimulation of Chemokine Receptors

As several retroviruses use chemokine receptors for virus entry, retroviral proteins may also contribute to pathogenesis by signaling cells through these chemokine receptors. For example, HIV-1 gp120-induced neuronal death can be inhibited by blocking or downregulating CXCR4 or CCR5 (Catani et al. 2000; Zhang et al. 2003; Zheng et al. 1999). CXCR4 expression has been detected on multiple cell types in the CNS including microglia, astrocytes, and neurons (Bajetto et al. 1999; Catani et al. 2000; Flynn et al. 2003), while CCR5 appears to be expressed on glial cells (van der Meer et al. 2000; Bajetto et al. 1999). Although HIV-1 primarily infects microglia/macrophages in the brain, HIV gp120-induced stimulation of CCR5 or CXCR4 may alter the activation state of uninfected cells or induce apoptosis. Another retroviral protein, Tat, is also reported to mimic chemokines. Tat acts as a chemoattractant to leukocytes, can induce CCL2(MCP-1) expression by astrocytes, and can displace the binding of a-chemokines from their receptors (Albini et al. 1998; Conant et al. 1998). HIV Tat also binds to the chemokine receptor CCR1 with similar affinity to the chemokine CCL7(MCP-3) (Albini et al. 1998), indicating that high levels of Tat may mimic the production of this chemokine.

The xenotropic/polytropic receptor 1 (XPR1, RMC1) is the cellular receptor for polytropic retrovirus infection (Tailor et al. 1999; Yang et al. 1999). Based on the presence of an SPX domain and similarities to the yeast protein SYG1, the XPR1 protein is predicted to be involved in G protein-associated signal transduction and function as a phosphate sensor (Battini et al. 1999). It is possible that XPR1 is involved in signal transduction of chemokine receptors or other signal transduction pathways that lead to the cellular activation. Further studies that elucidate the function of XPR1 would determine if stimulation of this receptor contributes to neuropathogenesis.

6
Conclusions

The correlation between increased proinflammatory cytokines and chemokines and neuropathogenesis induced by Fr98, HIV, SIV, and FIV suggests that some proinflammatory factors contribute to the disease process. Furthermore, polymorphism studies in HAD patients and knockout mouse studies in the Fr98 mouse model indicate that the upregulation of both TNF and CCL2(MCP-1) contributes to Fr98 and HIV-induced retroviral neuropathogenesis. Other proinflammatory cytokines, such as IL-1α or TNFSF1b(TNFβ, lymphotoxin A) may be a host reaction to retrovirus-induced damage. Proinflammatory cytokines and chemokines are most commonly known for their ability to recruit lymphocytes and other immune cells to the sites of infection. However, the upregulation of cytokines and chemokines associated with neuropathogenesis induced by HIV-1, SIV, FIV, and Fr98 retrovirus infection is not associated with substantial lymphocyte infiltration, possibly due to the immunosuppressed nature of the host. The pathogenesis of cytokines and chemokines during retrovirus infection may be due to stimulation of resident CNS cells. Several mechanisms by which proinflammatory cytokines and chemokines may contribute to the neuropathogenesis include the activation of perivascular macrophages and microglia, induction of neuronal apoptosis, interference with neuronal signal transduction, alteration of neuroprogenitor stem cell migration, and altering the activation and support functions of astrocytes. Further investigation is needed to determine the relative contribution of these mechanisms to the clinical neurological disorders associated with retrovirus infection. Additionally, it is important for possible therapeutic potential to determine whether certain chemokines might slow the progression of disease development as is suggested by some in vitro experiments.

References

Abbadie C, Lindia JA, Cumiskey AM, Peterson LB, Mudgett JS, Bayne EK, DeMartino JA, MacIntyre DE, Forrest MJ (2003) Impaired neuropathic pain responses in mice lacking the chemokine receptor CCR2. Proc Natl Acad Sci U S A 100:7947–7952

Adle-Biassette H, Chretien F, Wingertsmann L, Hery C, Ereau T, Scaravilli F, Tardieu M, Gray F (1999) Neuronal apoptosis does not correlate with dementia in HIV infection but is related to microglial activation and axonal damage. Neuropathol Appl Neurobiol 25:123–133

Albini A, Ferrini S, Benelli R, Sforzini S, Giunciuglio D, Aluigi MG, Proudfoot AE, Alouani S, Wells TN, Mariani G, Rabin RL, Farber JM, Noonan DM (1998) HIV-1 Tat protein mimicry of chemokines. Proc Natl Acad Sci U S A 95:13153–13158

Alkhatib G, Combadiere C, Broder CC, Feng Y, Kennedy PE, Murphy PM, Berger EA (1996) CC CKR5: a RANTES, MIP-1alpha, MIP-1beta receptor as a fusion cofactor for macrophage-tropic HIV-1. Science 272:1955–1958

Andjelkovic AV, Song L, Dzenko KA, Cong H, Pachter JS (2002) Functional expression of CCR2 by human fetal astrocytes. J Neurosci Res 70:219–231

Anthony IC, Ramage SN, Carnie FW, Simmonds P, Bell JE (2005) Influence of HAART on HIV-related CNS disease and neuroinflammation. J Neuropathol Exp Neurol 64:529–536

Araujo A, Hall WW (2004) Human T-lymphotropic virus type II and neurological disease. Ann Neurol 56:10–19

Asensio VC, Maier J, Milner R, Boztug K, Kincaid C, Moulard M, Phillipson C, Lindsley K, Krucker T, Fox HS, Campbell IL (2001) Interferon-independent, human immunodeficiency virus type 1 Gp120-mediated induction of CXCL10/IP-10 gene expression by astrocytes in vivo and in vitro. J Virol 75:7067–7077

Askovic S, Favara C, McAtee FJ, Portis JL (2001) Increased expression of MIP-1 alpha and MIP-1 beta mRNAs in the brain correlates spatially and temporally with the spongiform neurodegeneration induced by a murine oncornavirus. J Virol 75:2665–2674

Bagri A, Gurney T, He X, Zou YR, Littman DR, Tessier-Lavigne M, Pleasure SJ (2002) The chemokine SDF1 regulates migration of dentate granule cells. Development 129:4249–4260

Bajetto A, Bonavia R, Barbero S, Florio T, Costa A, Schettini G (1999) Expression of chemokine receptors in the rat brain. Ann N Y Acad Sci 876:201–209

Battini JL, Rasko JE, Miller AD (1999) A human cell-surface receptor for xenotropic and polytropic murine leukemia viruses: Possible role in G protein-coupled signal transduction. Proc Natl Acad Sci U S A 96:1385–1390

Boven LA, Middel J, Verhoef J, De Groot CJ, Nottet HS (2000) Monocyte infiltration is highly associated with loss of the tight junction protein Zonula occludens in HIV-1-associated dementia. Neuropathol Appl Neurobiol 26:356–360

Buller RS, Wehrly K, Portis JL, Chesebro B (1990) Host genes conferring resistance to a central nervous system disease induced by a polytropic recombinant friend murine retrovirus. J Virol 64:493–498

Catani MV, Corasaniti MT, Navarra M, Nistico G, Finazzi-Agro A, Melino G (2000) Gp120 Induces cell death in human neuroblastoma cells through the CXCR4 and CCR5 chemokine receptors. J Neurochem 74:2373–2379

Choe W, Stoica G, Lynn W, Wong PK (1998) Neurodegeneration induced by MoMuLV-Ts1 and increased expression of Fas and TNF-alpha in the central nervous system. Brain Res 779:1–8

Chretien F, Vallat-Decouvelaere AV, Bossuet C, Rimaniol AC, Le GR, Le PG, Creminon C, Dormont D, Gray F, Gras G (2002) Expression of excitatory amino acid transporter-2 (EAAT-2) and glutamine synthetase (GS) in brain macrophages and microglia of SIVmac251-infected macaques. Neuropathol Appl Neurobiol 28:410–417

Chretien F, Le PG, Vallat-Decouvelaere AV, Delisle MB, Uro-Coste E, Ironside JW, Gambetti P, Parchi P, Creminon C, Dormont D, Mikol J, Gray F, Gras G (2004) Expression of excitatory amino acid transporter-1 (EAAT-1) in brain macrophages and microglia of patients with prion diseases. J Neuropathol Exp Neurol 63:1058–1071

Christensen T (2005) Association of human endogenous retroviruses with multiple sclerosis and possible interactions with herpes viruses. Rev Med Virol 15:179–211

Conant K, Garzino-Demo A, Nath A, McArthur JC, Halliday W, Power C, Gallo RC, Major EO (1998) Induction of monocyte chemoattractant protein-1 in HIV-1 Tat-stimulated astrocytes and elevation in AIDS dementia. Proc Natl Acad Sci U S A 95:3117–3121

Croitoru-Lamoury J, Guillemin GJ, Boussin FD, Mognetti B, Gigout LI, Cheret A, Vaslin B, Le GR, Brew BJ, Dormont D (2003) Expression of chemokines and their receptors in human and Simian astrocytes: evidence for a central role of TNF alpha and IFN gamma in CXCR4 and CCR5 modulation. Glia 41:354–370

Czub M, McAtee FJ, Czub S, Lynch WP, Portis JL (1995) Prevention of retrovirus-induced neurological disease by infection with a nonneuropathogenic retrovirus. Virology 206:372–380

Dimcheff DE, Askovic S, Baker AH, Johnson-Fowler C, Portis JL (2003) Endoplasmic reticulum stress is a determinant of retrovirus-induced spongiform neurodegeneration. J Virol 77:12617–12629

Dimcheff DE, Faasse MA, McAtee FJ, Portis JL (2004) Endoplasmic reticulum (ER) stress induced by a neurovirulent mouse retrovirus is associated with prolonged BiP binding and retention of a viral protein in the ER. J Biol Chem 279:33782–33790

Dorf ME, Berman MA, Tanabe S, Heesen M, Luo Y (2000) Astrocytes express functional chemokine receptors. J Neuroimmunol 111:109–121

Drapeau E, Mayo W, Aurousseau C, Le MM, Piazza PV, Abrous DN (2003) Spatial memory performances of aged rats in the water maze predict levels of hippocampal neurogenesis. Proc Natl Acad Sci U S A 100:14385–14390

Dufour JH, Dziejman M, Liu MT, Leung JH, Lane TE, Luster AD (2002) IFN-gamma-inducible protein 10 (IP-10; CXCL10)-deficient mice reveal a role for IP-10 in effector T cell generation and trafficking. J Immunol 168:3195–3204

Dzenko KA, Song L, Ge S, Kuziel WA, Pachter JS (2005) CCR2 expression by brain microvascular endothelial cells is critical for macrophage transendothelial migration in response to CCL2. Microvasc Res [Epub ahead of print]

Eugenin EA, Berman JW (2003) Chemokine-dependent mechanisms of leukocyte trafficking across a model of the blood-brain barrier. Methods 29:351–361

Eugenin EA, D'Aversa TG, Lopez L, Calderon TM, Berman JW (2003) MCP-1 (CCL2) Protects human neurons and astrocytes From NMDA or HIV-Tat-induced apoptosis. J Neurochem 85:1299–1311

Feng Y, Broder CC, Kennedy PE, Berger EA (1996) HIV-1 entry cofactor: functional cDNA cloning of a seven-transmembrane, G protein-coupled receptor. Science 272:872–877

Flynn G, Maru S, Loughlin J, Romero IA, Male D (2003) Regulation of chemokine receptor expression in human microglia and astrocytes. J Neuroimmunol 136:84–93

Gardner MB (1988) Neurotropic retroviruses of wild mice and macaques. Ann Neurol 23 Suppl:S201–S206

Gardner MB, Dandekar S (1995) Neurobiology of simian and feline immunodeficiency virus infections. Curr Top Microbiol Immunol 202:135–150

Gardner MB, Henderson BE, Officer JE, Rongey RW, Parker JC, Oliver C, Estes JD, Huebner RJ (1973) A spontaneous lower motor neuron disease apparently caused by indigenous type-C RNA virus in wild mice. J Natl Cancer Inst 51:1243–1254

Georgsson G (1994) Neuropathologic aspects of lentiviral infections. Ann N Y Acad Sci 724:50–67

Glabinski A, Krajewski S, Rafalowska J (1998) Tumor necrosis factor-alpha induced pathology in the rat brain: characterization of stereotaxic injection model. Folia Neuropathol 36:52–62

Glass JD, Wesselingh SL, Selnes OA, McArthur JC (1993) Clinical-neuropathologic correlation in HIV-associated dementia [see comments]. Neurology 43:2230–2237

Glass JD, Fedor H, Wesselingh SL, McArthur JC (1995) Immunocytochemical quantitation of human immunodeficiency virus in the brain: correlations with dementia. Ann Neurol 38:755–762

Gonzalez E, Rovin BH, Sen L, Cooke G, Dhanda R, Mummidi S, Kulkarni H, Bamshad MJ, Telles V, Anderson SA, Walter EA, Stephan KT, Deucher M, Mangano A, Bologna R, Ahuja SS, Dolan MJ, Ahuja SK (2002) HIV-1 infection and AIDS dementia are influenced by a mutant MCP-1 allele linked to increased monocyte infiltration of tissues and MCP-1 levels. Proc Natl Acad Sci U S A 99:13795–13800

Gorry PR, Bristol G, Zack JA, Ritola K, Swanstrom R, Birch CJ, Bell JE, Bannert N, Crawford K, Wang H, Schols D, De CE, Kunstman K, Wolinsky SM, Gabuzda D (2001) Macrophage tropism of human immunodeficiency virus type 1 isolates from brain and lymphoid tissues predicts neurotropism independent of coreceptor specificity. J Virol 75:10073–10089

Guo H, Lai L, Butchbach ME, Stockinger MP, Shan X, Bishop GA, Lin CL (2003) Increased expression of the glial glutamate transporter EAAT2 modulates excitotoxicity and delays the onset but not the outcome of ALS in mice. Hum Mol Genet 12:2519–2532

Guyon A, Rovere C, Cervantes A, Allaeys I, Nahon JL (2005) Stromal cell-derived factor-1alpha directly modulates voltage-dependent currents of the action potential in mammalian neuronal cells. J Neurochem 93:963–973

Haase AT (1986) Pathogenesis of lentivirus infections. Nature 322:130–136

Hasenkrug KJ, Robertson SJ, Porti J, McAtee F, Nishio J, Chesebro B (1996) Two separate envelope regions influence induction of brain disease by a polytropic murine retrovirus (FMCF98). J Virol 70:4825–4828

Hoffman PM, Cimino EF, Robbins DS, Broadwell RD, Powers JM, Ruscetti SK (1992) Cellular tropism and localization in the rodent nervous system of a neuropathogenic variant of friend murine leukemia virus. Lab Invest 67:314–321

Humbles AA, Lu B, Friend DS, Okinaga S, Lora J, Al-Garawi A, Martin TR, Gerard NP, Gerard C (2002) The murine CCR3 receptor regulates both the role of eosinophils and mast cells in allergen-induced airway inflammation and hyperresponsiveness. Proc Natl Acad Sci U S A 99:1479–1484

Hurwitz AA, Berman JW, Lyman WD (1994) The role of the blood-brain barrier in HIV infection of the central nervous system. Adv Neuroimmunol 4:249–256

Jacobson S (2002) Immunopathogenesis of human T cell lymphotropic virus type I-associated neurologic disease. J Infect Dis 186 Suppl 2:S187–S192

Johnston JB, Silva C, Hiebert T, Buist R, Dawood MR, Peeling J, Power C (2002) Neurovirulence depends on virus input titer in brain in feline immunodeficiency virus infection: evidence for activation of innate immunity and neuronal injury. J Neurovirol 8:420–431

Jolicoeur P, Hu C, Mak TW, Martinou JC, Kay DG (2003) Protection against murine leukemia virus-induced spongiform myeloencephalopathy in mice overexpressing Bcl-2 but not in mice deficient for interleukin-6, inducible nitric oxide synthetase, ICE, Fas, Fas ligand, or TNF-R1 genes. J Virol 77:13161–13170

Kai K, Furuta T (1984) Isolation of paralysis-inducing murine leukemia viruses from friend virus passaged in rats. J Virol 50:970–973

Khan IA, Murphy PM, Casciotti L, Schwartzman JD, Collins J, Gao JL, Yeaman GR (2001) Mice lacking the chemokine receptor CCR1 show increased susceptibility to Toxoplasma gondii infection. J Immunol 166:1930–1937

Kim HT, Waters K, Stoica G, Qiang W, Liu N, Scofield VL, Wong PK (2004a) Activation of endoplasmic reticulum stress signaling pathway is associated with neuronal degeneration in MoMuLV-Ts1-induced spongiform encephalomyelopathy. Lab Invest 84:816–827

Kim WK, Corey S, Chesney G, Knight H, Klumpp S, Wuthrich C, Letvin N, Koralnik I, Lackner A, Veasey R, Williams K (2004b) Identification of T lymphocytes in simian immunodeficiency virus encephalitis: distribution of CD8$^+$ T cells in association with central nervous system vessels and virus. J Neurovirol 10:315–325

Kolb SA, Sporer B, Lahrtz F, Koedel U, Pfister HW, Fontana A (1999) Identification of a T cell chemotactic factor in the cerebrospinal fluid of HIV-1-infected individuals as interferon-gamma inducible protein 10. J Neuroimmunol 93:172–181

Kolson DL, Lavi E, Gonzalez-Scarano F (1998) The effects of human immunodeficiency virus in the central nervous system. Adv Virus Res 50:1–47

Krathwohl MD, Kaiser JL (2004) HIV-1 promotes quiescence in human neural progenitor cells. J Infect Dis 190:216–226

Kutsch O, Oh J, Nath A, Benveniste EN (2000) Induction of the chemokines interleukin-8 and IP-10 by human immunodeficiency virus type 1 Tat in astrocytes. J Virol 74:9214–9221

Kuziel WA, Morgan SJ, Dawson TC, Griffin S, Smithies O, Ley K, Maeda N (1997) Severe reduction in leukocyte adhesion and monocyte extravasation in mice deficient in CC chemokine receptor 2. Proc Natl Acad Sci U S A 94:12053–12058

Kuziel WA, Dawson TC, Quinones M, Garavito E, Chenaux G, Ahuja SS, Reddick RL, Maeda N (2003) CCR5 deficiency is not protective in the early stages of atherogenesis in ApoE knockout mice. Atherosclerosis 167:25–32

Lackner AA, Dandekar S, Gardner MB (1991) Neurobiology of simian and feline immunodeficiency virus infections. Brain Pathol 1:201–212

Lane TE, Buchmeier MJ, Watry DD, Fox HS (1996) Expression of inflammatory cytokines and inducible nitric oxide synthase in brains of SIV-infected rhesus monkeys: applications to HIV-induced central nervous system disease. Mol Med 2:27–37

Li S, Mallory M, Alford M, Tanaka S, Masliah E (1997) Glutamate transporter alterations in Alzheimer disease are possibly associated with abnormal APP expression. J Neuropathol Exp Neurol 56:901–911

Liberto CM, Albrecht PJ, Herx LM, Yong VW, Levison SW (2004) Pro-regenerative properties of cytokine-activated astrocytes. J Neurochem 89:1092–1100

Liu N, Kuang X, Kim HT, Stoica G, Qiang W, Scofield VL, Wong PK (2004) Possible involvement of both endoplasmic reticulum- and mitochondria-dependent pathways in MoMuLV-Ts1-induced apoptosis in astrocytes. J Neurovirol 10:189–198

Lu B, Rutledge BJ, Gu L, Fiorillo J, Lukacs NW, Kunkel SL, North R, Gerard C, Rollins BJ (1998) Abnormalities in monocyte recruitment and cytokine expression in monocyte chemoattractant protein 1-deficient mice. J Exp Med 187:601–608

Lu M, Grove EA, Miller RJ (2002) Abnormal development of the hippocampal dentate gyrus in mice lacking the CXCR4 chemokine receptor. Proc Natl Acad Sci U S A 99:7090–7095

Luabeya MK, Dallasta LM, Achim CL, Pauza CD, Hamilton RL (2000) Blood-brain barrier disruption in simian immunodeficiency virus encephalitis. Neuropathol Appl Neurobiol 26:454–462

Lynch WP, Czub S, McAtee FJ, Hayes SF, Portis JL (1991) Murine retrovirus-induced spongiform encephalopathy: productive infection of microglia and cerebellar neurons in accelerated CNS disease. Neuron 7:365–379

Margulies BJ, Hauer DA, Clements JE (2001) Identification and comparison of eleven rhesus macaque chemokine receptors. AIDS Res Hum Retroviruses 17:981–986

Martin LJ, Price AC, Kaiser A, Shaikh AY, Liu Z (2000) Mechanisms for neuronal degeneration in amyotrophic lateral sclerosis and in models of motor neuron death (review). Int J Mol Med 5:3–13

McManus CM, Weidenheim K, Woodman SE, Nunez J, Hesselgesser J, Nath A, Berman JW (2000) Chemokine and chemokine-receptor expression in human glial elements: induction by the HIV protein, Tat, and chemokine autoregulation. Am J Pathol 156:1441–1453

Meucci O, Fatatis A, Simen AA, Bushell TJ, Gray PW, Miller RJ (1998) Chemokines regulate hippocampal neuronal signaling and Gp120 neurotoxicity. Proc Natl Acad Sci U S A 95:14500–14505

Miller RF, Isaacson PG, Hall-Craggs M, Lucas S, Gray F, Scaravilli F, An SF (2004) Cerebral CD8+ lymphocytosis in HIV-1 infected patients with immune restoration induced by HAART. Acta Neuropathol (Berl) 108:17–23

Monje ML, Toda H, Palmer TD (2003) Inflammatory blockade restores adult hippocampal neurogenesis. Science 302:1760–1765

Moser B, Wolf M, Walz A, Loetscher P (2004) Chemokines: multiple levels of leukocyte migration control. Trends Immunol 25:75–84

Murphy SL, Honczarenko MJ, Dugger NV, Hoffman PM, Gaulton GN (2004) Disparate regions of envelope protein regulate syncytium formation versus spongiform encephalopathy in neurological disease induced by murine leukemia virus TR. J Virol 78:8392–8399

Nukuna A, Gendelman H, Limoges J, Rasmussen J, Poluektova L, Ghorpade A, Persidsky Y (2004) Levels of human immunodeficiency virus type 1 (HIV-1) replication in macrophages determines the severity of murine HIV-1 encephalitis. J Neurovirol 10:82–90

Oaks JL, Long MT, Baszler TV (2004) Leukoencephalitis associated with selective viral replication in the brain of a pony with experimental chronic equine infectious anemia virus infection. Vet Pathol 41:527–532

Oberlin E, Amara A, Bachelerie F, Bessia C, Virelizier JL, renzana-Seisdedos F, Schwartz O, Heard JM, Clark-Lewis I, Legler DF, Loetscher M, Baggiolini M, Moser B (1996) The CXC chemokine SDF-1 is the ligand for LESTR/Fusin and prevents infection by T-cell-line-adapted HIV-1. Nature 382:833–835

Orandle MS, MacLean AG, Sasseville VG, Alvarez X, Lackner AA (2002) Enhanced expression of proinflammatory cytokines in the central nervous system is associated with neuroinvasion by simian immunodeficiency virus and the development of encephalitis. J Virol 76:5797–5802

Park BH, Lavi E, Blank KJ, Gaulton GN (1993) Intracerebral hemorrhages and syncytium formation induced by endothelial cell infection with a murine leukemia virus. J Virol 67:6015–6024

Park BH, Lavi E, Stieber A, Gaulton GN (1994) Pathogenesis of cerebral infarction and hemorrhage induced by a murine leukemia virus. Lab Invest 70:78–85

Patrick MK, Johnston JB, Power C (2002) Lentiviral neuropathogenesis: comparative neuroinvasion, neurotropism, neurovirulence, and host neurosusceptibility. J Virol 76:7923–7931

Persidsky Y, Ghorpade A, Rasmussen J, Limoges J, Liu XJ, Stins M, Fiala M, Way D, Kim KS, Witte MH, Weinand M, Carhart L, Gendelman HE (1999) Microglial and astrocyte chemokines regulate monocyte migration through the blood-brain barrier in human immunodeficiency virus-1 encephalitis. Am J Pathol 155:1599–1611

Peterson KE, Robertson SJ, Portis JL, Chesebro B (2001) Differences in cytokine and chemokine responses during neurological disease induced by polytropic murine retroviruses map to separate regions of the viral envelope gene. J Virol 75:2848–2856

Peterson KE, Errett JS, Wei T, Dimcheff DE, Ransohoff R, Kuziel WA, Evans L, Chesebro B (2004a) MCP-1 and CCR2 contribute to non-lymphocyte-mediated brain disease induced by Fr98 polytropic retrovirus infection in mice: role for astrocytes in retroviral neuropathogenesis. J Virol 78:6449–6458

Peterson KE, Hughes S, Dimcheff DE, Wehrly K, Chesebro B (2004b) Separate sequences in a murine retroviral envelope protein mediate neuropathogenesis by complementary mechanisms with differing requirements for tumor necrosis factor alpha. J Virol 78:13104–13112

Petito CK, Adkins B, McCarthy M, Roberts B, Khamis I (2003) $CD4^+$ and $CD8^+$ cells accumulate in the brains of acquired immunodeficiency syndrome patients with human immunodeficiency virus encephalitis. J Neurovirol 9:36–44

Poli A, Abramo F, Di Iorio C, Cantile C, Carli MA, Pollera C, Vago L, Tosoni A, Costanzi G (1997) Neuropathology in cats experimentally infected with feline immunodeficiency virus: a morphological, immunocytochemical and morphometric study. J Neurovirol 3:361–368

Poli A, Pistello M, Carli MA, Abramo F, Mancuso G, Nicoletti E, Bendinelli M (1999) Tumor necrosis factor-alpha and virus expression in the central nervous system of cats infected with feline immunodeficiency virus. J Neurovirol 5:465–473

Portis JL (2001) Genetic determinants of neurovirulence of murine oncornaviruses. Adv Virus Res 56:3–38

Portis JL, Czub S, Robertson S, McAtee F, Chesebro B (1995) Characterization of a neurologic disease induced by a polytropic murine retrovirus: evidence for differential targeting of ecotropic and polytropic viruses in the brain. J Virol 69:8070–8075

Potash MJ, Chao W, Bentsman G, Paris N, Saini M, Nitkiewicz J, Belem P, Sharer L, Brooks AI, Volsky DJ (2005) A mouse model for study of systemic HIV-1 infection, antiviral immune responses, and neuroinvasiveness. Proc Natl Acad Sci U S A 102:3760–3765

Poulsen DJ, Robertson SJ, Favara CA, Portis JL, Chesebro BW (1998) mapping of a neurovirulence determinant within the envelope protein of a polytropic murine retrovirus: induction of central nervous system disease by low levels of virus. Virology 248:199–207

Poulsen DJ, Favara C, Snyder EY, Portis J, Chesebro B (1999) Increased neurovirulence of polytropic mouse retroviruses delivered by inoculation of brain with infected neural stem cells. Virology 263:23–29

Power C, Johnson RT (1995) HIV-1 associated dementia: clinical features and pathogenesis. Can J Neurol Sci 22:92–100

Power C, Johnson RT (2001) Neuroimmune and neurovirological aspects of human immunodeficiency virus infection. Adv Virus Res 56:389–433

Power C, Zhang K, Van Marle G (2004) Comparative neurovirulence in lentiviral infections: the roles of viral molecular diversity and select proteases. J Neurovirol 10 Suppl 1:113–117

Quasney MW, Zhang Q, Sargent S, Mynatt M, Glass J, McArthur J (2001) Increased frequency of the tumor necrosis factor-alpha-308 A allele in adults with human immunodeficiency virus dementia. Ann Neurol 50:157–162

Ransohoff RM (2002) The chemokine system in neuroinflammation: an update. J Infect Dis 186 Suppl 2:S152–S156

Ransohoff RM, Tani M (1998) Do chemokines mediate leukocyte recruitment in posttraumatic CNS inflammation? Trends Neurosci 21:154–159

Rausch DM, Heyes MP, Murray EA, Lendvay J, Sharer LR, Ward JM, Rehm S, Nohr D, Weihe E, Eiden LE (1994) Cytopathologic and neurochemical correlates of progression to motor/cognitive impairment in SIV-infected rhesus monkeys. J Neuropathol Exp Neurol 53:165–175

Robertson SJ, Hasenkrug KJ, Chesebro B, Portis JL (1997) Neurologic disease induced by polytropic murine retroviruses: neurovirulence determined by efficiency of spread to microglial cells. J Virol 71:5287–5294

Rola R, Raber J, Rizk A, Otsuka S, VandenBerg SR, Morhardt DR, Fike JR (2004) Radiation-induced impairment of hippocampal neurogenesis is associated with cognitive deficits in young mice. Exp Neurol 188:316–330

Saha RN, Pahan K (2003) Tumor necrosis factor-alpha at the crossroads of neuronal life and death during HIV-associated dementia. J Neurochem 86:1057–1071

Sasseville VG, Smith MM, Mackay CR, Pauley DR, Mansfield KG, Ringler DJ, Lackner AA (1996) Chemokine expression in simian immunodeficiency virus-induced AIDS encephalitis. Am J Pathol 149:1459–1467

Schmidtmayerova H, Nottet HS, Nuovo G, Raabe T, Flanagan CR, Dubrovsky L, Gendelman HE, Cerami A, Bukrinsky M, Sherry B (1996) Human immunodeficiency virus type 1 infection alters chemokine beta peptide expression in human monocytes: implications for recruitment of leukocytes into brain and lymph nodes. Proc Natl Acad Sci U S A 93:700–704

Sigurdsson B, Palsson P, Grimsson H (1957) Visna, a demyelinating transmissible disease of sheep. J Neuropathol Exp Neurol 16:389–403

Sigurdsson B, Thormar H, Palsson P (1960) Cultivation of visna virus in tissue culture. Arch Gesamte Virusforsch 10:368–381

Sopper S, Demuth M, Stahl-Hennig C, Hunsmann G, Plesker R, Coulibaly C, Czub S, Ceska M, Koutsilieri E, Riederer P, Brinkmann R, Katz M, ter Meulen V (1996) The effect of simian immunodeficiency virus infection in vitro and in vivo on the cytokine production of isolated microglia and peripheral macrophages from rhesus monkey. Virology 220:320–329

Sui Y, Potula R, Pinson D, Adany I, Li Z, Day J, Buch E, Segebrecht J, Villinger F, Liu Z, Huang M, Narayan O, Buch S (2003) Microarray analysis of cytokine and chemokine genes in the brains of macaques with SHIV-encephalitis. J Med Primatol 32:229–239

Tailor CS, Nouri A, Lee CG, Kozak C, Kabat D (1999) Cloning and characterization of a cell surface receptor for xenotropic and polytropic murine leukemia viruses. Proc Natl Acad Sci U S A 96:927–932

Tanabe S, Heesen M, Berman MA, Fischer MB, Yoshizawa I, Luo Y, Dorf ME (1997) Murine astrocytes express a functional chemokine receptor. J Neurosci 17:6522–6528

Tran PB, Miller RJ (2003) Chemokine receptors: signposts to brain development and disease. Nat Rev Neurosci 4:444–455

Tran PB, Ren D, Veldhouse TJ, Miller RJ (2004) Chemokine receptors are expressed widely by embryonic and adult neural progenitor cells. J Neurosci Res 76:20–34

Tyor WR, Glass JD, Griffin JW, Becker PS, McArthur JC, Bezman L, Griffin DE (1992) Cytokine expression in the brain during the acquired immunodeficiency syndrome. Ann Neurol 31:349–360

Vago L, Nebuloni M, Bonetto S, Pellegrinelli A, Zerbi P, Ferri A, Lavri E, Capra M, Grassi MP, Costanzi G (2001) Rantes distribution and cellular localization in the brain of HIV-infected patients. Clin Neuropathol 20:139–145

van der Meer P, Ulrich AM, Gonzalez-Scarano F, Lavi E (2000) Immunohistochemical analysis of CCR2, CCR3, CCR5, and CXCR4 in the human brain: potential mechanisms for HIV dementia. Exp Mol Pathol 69:192–201

van Gassen KL, Netzeband JG, de Graan PN, Gruol DL (2005) The Chemokine CCL2 modulates Ca dynamics and electrophysiological properties of cultured cerebellar Purkinje neurons. Eur J Neurosci 21:2949–2957

van Rij RP, Portegies P, Hallaby T, Lange JM, Visser J, de Roda Husman AM, van't Wout AB, Schuitemaker H (1999) Reduced prevalence of the CCR5 delta32 heterozygous genotype in human immunodeficiency virus-infected individuals with AIDS dementia complex. J Infect Dis 180:854–857

Wang EJ, Sun J, Pettoello-Mantovani M, Anderson CM, Osiecki K, Zhao ML, Lopez L, Lee SC, Berman JW, Goldstein H (2003) Microglia from mice transgenic for a provirus encoding a monocyte-tropic HIV type 1 isolate produce infectious virus and display in vitro and in vivo upregulation of lipopolysaccharide-induced chemokine gene expression. AIDS Res Hum Retroviruses 19:755–765

Widera D, Holtkamp W, Entschladen F, Niggemann B, Zanker K, Kaltschmidt B, Kaltschmidt C (2004) MCP-1 induces migration of adult neural stem cells. Eur J Cell Biol 83:381–387

Williams K, Alvarez X, Lackner AA (2001) Central nervous system perivascular cells are immunoregulatory cells that connect the CNS with the peripheral immune system. Glia 36:156–164

Williams KC, Hickey WF (2002) Central nervous system damage, monocytes and macrophages, and neurological disorders in AIDS. Annu Rev Neurosci 25:537–562

Wong PK, Knupp C, Yuen PH, Soong MM, Zachary JF, Tompkins WA (1985) Ts1, a paralytogenic mutant of Moloney murine leukemia virus TB, has an enhanced ability to replicate in the central nervous system and primary nerve cell culture. J Virol 55:760–767

Yang YL, Guo L, Xu S, Holland CA, Kitamura T, Hunter K, Cunningham JM (1999) Receptors for polytropic and xenotropic mouse leukaemia viruses encoded by a single gene at Rmc1. Nat Genet 21:216–219

Zhang K, Rana F, Silva C, Ethier J, Wehrly K, Chesebro B, Power C (2003) Human immunodeficiency virus type 1 envelope-mediated neuronal death: uncoupling of viral replication and neurotoxicity. J Virol 77:6899–6912

Zheng J, Ghorpade A, Niemann D, Cotter RL, Thylin MR, Epstein L, Swartz JM, Shepard RB, Liu X, Nukuna A, Gendelman HE (1999) Lymphotropic virions affect chemokine receptor-mediated neural signaling and apoptosis: implications for human immunodeficiency virus type 1-associated dementia. J Virol 73:8256–8267

Zink MC, Coleman GD, Mankowski JL, Adams RJ, Tarwater PM, Fox K, Clements JE (2001) Increased macrophage chemoattractant protein-1 in cerebrospinal fluid precedes and predicts simian immunodeficiency virus encephalitis. J Infect Dis 184:1015–1021

HIV-1 Coreceptors and Their Inhibitors

N. Ray (✉) · R. W. Doms

Department of Microbiology, University of Pennsylvania, 301A Johnson Pavilion, Philadelphia, PA 19104, USA
nray@mail.med.upenn.edu

1	Identification of Chemokine Receptors as Coreceptors for HIV-1 Env-Mediated Fusion	98
2	Determinants of Tropism and Chemokine Receptor Usage	101
3	Impact of Nonfunctional Chemokine Receptor Alleles on HIV-1 Resistance and Disease Progression	101
4	Coreceptor-Based Antiretroviral Therapy	103
4.1	CCR5-Based Antiretroviral Therapy	103
4.1.1	TAK-779, TAK-220, and TAK-652	104
4.1.2	SCH-C and SCH-D	105
4.1.3	UK-427857 (Maraviroc)	106
4.1.4	CMPD 167	106
4.1.5	Spirodiketopiperazine-Based Inhibitors	107
4.2	CXCR4-Based Antiretroviral Therapy	107
4.2.1	Small Molecule CXCR4 Inhibitors	107
5	Resistance to Coreceptor Inhibitors	108
6	Impact of Chemokine Receptor Inhibitors on Clinical Monitoring and Treatment	109
	References	110

Abstract Entry of human immunodeficiency virus (HIV) into target cells is mediated by the viral Envelope glycoprotein (Env) and its coordinated interaction with a receptor (CD4) and a coreceptor (usually the chemokine receptors CCR5 or CXCR4). This review describes the identification of chemokine receptors as coreceptors for HIV-1 Env-mediated fusion, the determinants of chemokine receptor usage, and the impact of nonfunctional chemokine receptor alleles on HIV-1 resistance and disease progression. Due to the important role of chemokine receptors in HIV-1 entry, inhibitors of these coreceptors are good candidates for blocking entry and development of antiretroviral therapies. We discuss the different CCR5- and CXCR4-based antiretroviral drugs that have been developed thus far, highlighting the most promising drug candidates. Resistance to these coreceptor inhibitors as well as the impact of these drugs on clinical monitoring and treatment are also discussed.

1
Identification of Chemokine Receptors as Coreceptors for HIV-1 Env-Mediated Fusion

Human immunodeficiency virus (HIV) initiates infection by attaching and subsequently fusing its viral membrane to the plasma membrane of a target cell. As shown in Fig. 1, the process is mediated primarily by the viral Envelope protein (Env). Env is a glycoprotein, 160 kDa in size (gp160), that is proteolytically processed into a surface subunit (gp120) and a transmembrane subunit (gp41) by a host cell protease during transit to the cell surface. Each gp120 molecule interacts with one gp41 molecule to form a noncovalently linked complex, and the gp120–gp41 complexes then exist as trimers on the surface of HIV virions. These trimers bind with high affinity to CD4, the primary receptor for HIV on the target cell surface. The presence of CD4 is a prerequisite for efficient HIV infection and explains the tropism of HIV for CD4-positive T cells and macrophages.

Three main lines of evidence derived from experiments reported in the mid-1980s and early 1990s, however, brought into question the role of CD4 as the only receptor for HIV. First, studies with recombinant human CD4 demonstrated the ability of this molecule to render cells susceptible to Env-mediated fusion and virus entry, but only when expressed in human cell types [20, 61]. Further work with cell hybrids pointed toward the existence of an essential coreceptor, specific to human cells, in the absence of which CD4 was unable to support Env-mediated fusion [4, 14]. Second, in the late 1980s, different HIV-1 isolates were shown to display distinct tropisms for various

Fig. 1 Model of HIV entry. The Env glycoprotein of HIV mediates fusion of viral and cellular membranes. Env is a homotrimeric protein (*first panel*) in which each subunit is composed of surface gp120 and membrane-spanning gp41 proteins. Binding to CD4 is mediated by the gp120 subunit, and CD4 binding induces conformational changes in gp120 that result in the exposure of a conserved region that is important for coreceptor binding (*second panel*). In the native trimer, this conserved region is hidden in part by variable loops that are thought to undergo conformational changes and consequent repositioning after CD4 binding. Following CD4 binding, gp120 binds to a seven-transmembrane domain coreceptor (CoR; *third panel*). Coreceptor binding can be inhibited by a number of CCR5 and CXCR4 inhibitors such as TAK-220, SCH-C, SCH-D, UK-427,857, CMPD 167, GSK-873140, AMD-3100, and AMD-070. The hydrophobic fusion peptide at the N terminus of gp41 becomes exposed and inserts into the cell membrane. Ultimately, coreceptor binding leads to the formation of a six-helix bundle in which the helical HR2 domains of each gp41 subunit fold back and bind to the triple-stranded HR1 domains (*fourth panel*), bringing the fusion peptide and transmembrane domain of gp41, and their associated membranes, into close proximity

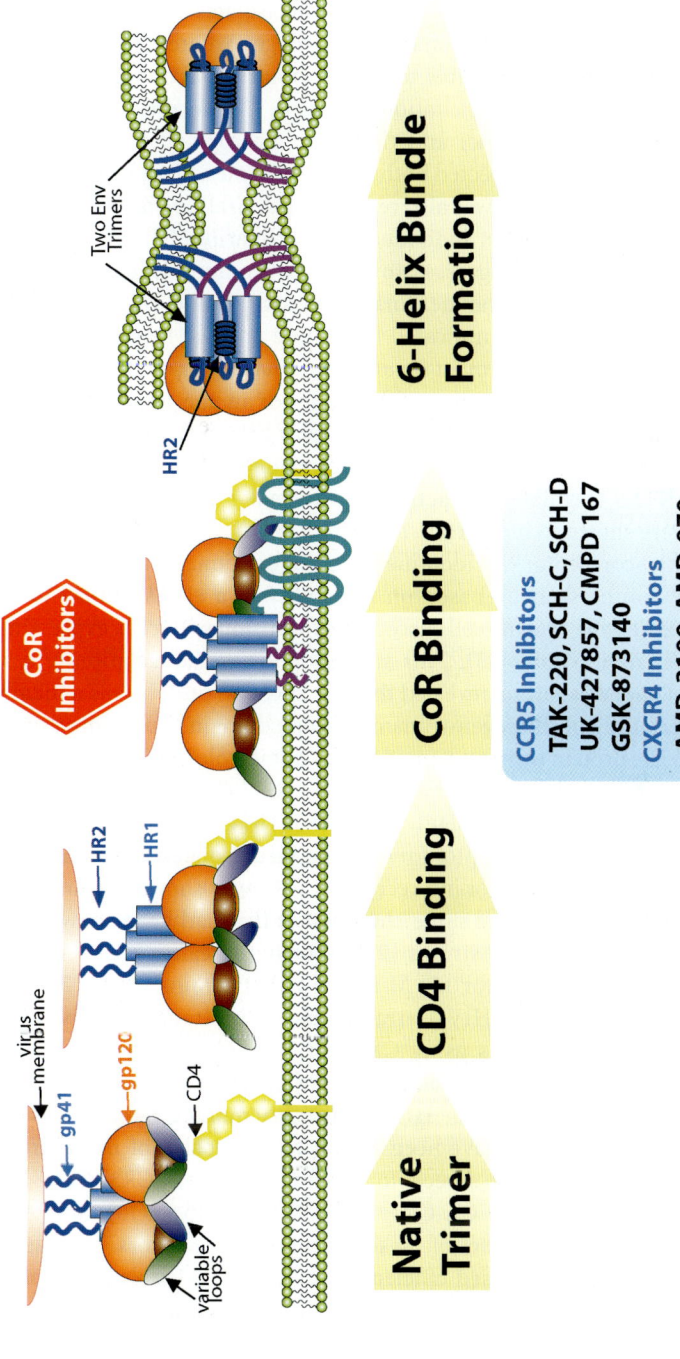

CD4-positive human cell types in vitro. Some isolates are able to infect CD4-positive T cell lines but not primary macrophages, whereas others showed the opposite tropism and were able to infect primary macrophages much better than T cell lines ([71] and citations therein). The former were designated T cell-line tropic (T-tropic) and the latter macrophage tropic (M-tropic). Isolates that efficiently infected both T cell lines and macrophages were called dual-tropic. Soon after, it was also reported that viral isolates from peripheral blood of recently infected individuals are primarily M-tropic [85, 91, 116] and as the infection progresses to acquired immunodeficiency syndrome (AIDS), T-tropic viruses can be isolated in most patients [23, 91, 102]. Again, cell hybrid experiments indicated that these specific tropisms were likely resulting from the requirement for an additional coreceptor in the susceptible cells rather than the presence of an inhibitor in the nonsusceptible cells. Finally, the identity of the putative coreceptor became apparent from studies with the chemokines macrophage inflammatory protein (MIP)-1α, MIP-1β, and RANTES (regulated on activation, normal T-expressed and secreted), which were shown to block HIV-1 infection [21].

The first coreceptor was identified using a functional complementary DNA (cDNA) cloning strategy based on the ability of a cDNA library to render a CD4-expressing murine cell susceptible for fusion with cells expressing Env from a T-tropic strain [43]. This strategy allowed the isolation of a single cDNA; sequence analysis revealed that the encoded protein was a member of the superfamily of the seven-transmembrane domain G protein-coupled receptors. The protein was first named "fusin" for its role in HIV fusion, and later CXCR4 when it was shown to be a chemokine receptor for the CXC chemokines stromal cell-derived factor (SDF)-1α and SDF-1β [11, 78]. Importantly, CXCR4 did not function as a coreceptor for M-tropic virus isolates. However, at around the same time, the chemokine receptor CCR5 was shown to bind MIP-1α, MIP-1β, and RANTES, the same chemokines that had been shown to block infection by some HIV-1 strains [21]. Shortly thereafter, CCR5 was shown to be the major coreceptor for M-tropic HIV-1 strains [3, 19, 32, 37, 39]. CCR5-using (R5-tropic) HIV-1 strains tend to be transmitted between individuals, whereas strains using CXCR4 (X4-tropic) emerge in a subset of HIV-1-infected individuals at later stages of infection [25, 96]. In addition to the two main coreceptors for HIV-1, other chemokine receptors as well as some orphan receptors have been shown to be capable of mediating virus fusion. These alternative coreceptors include CCR2b, CCR3, CCR8, CCR9, CXCR6 (STRL33/Bonzo), CX_3CR1, ChemR23, GPR15 (BOB), and APJ (reviewed in [8, 95]). A subset of these alternative coreceptors, such as CCR3, CCR8, and CXCR6, are used efficiently by some HIV-1 isolates to infect cell lines over-expressing these proteins [7, 86, 114]. Certain minor coreceptors

(CXCR6 and GPR15) are expressed in the placenta and colon and could conceivably play a role in mother-to-child or homosexual transmission [33], while CCR8 is expressed on thymocytes and so could play a role in virus infection in the thymus. However, with only a handful of exceptions [93, 110, 115], infection of human macrophages and peripheral blood mononuclear cells (PBMCs) by HIV-1 strains is dependent upon the presence of either CCR5 or CXCR4 in conjunction with CD4. Most of the alternative coreceptors are either not expressed on CD4-positive cells at detectable levels, or are expressed at levels that are below that needed for efficient virus infection. Thus, at present there is no compelling evidence to indicate that receptors other than CCR5 or CXCR4 are important for HIV-1 infection in vivo.

2
Determinants of Tropism and Chemokine Receptor Usage

The *env* genes from different HIV-1 isolates display significant sequence heterogeneity in specific regions of gp120. There are five variable regions in gp120 (V1–V5) that are separated by five constant regions (C1–C5). Studies involving Env chimeras between M- and T-tropic isolates identified the V3 loop as the primary determinant of viral tropism [17, 18, 28, 51, 94, 101] and coreceptor usage [19, 22, 85, 98, 99]. Although even single amino acid changes in the V3 loop have been shown to be sufficient to alter tropism [27], many of the mutations observed in this region that alter tropism have strain-specific effects, and no single amino acid has emerged as crucial. In general, however, an increase in the net positive charge (i.e., more basic residues) in the V3 loop has been demonstrated in viral isolates from HIV-positive patients over time and correlates with conversion to T cell tropism and CXCR4 usage [9, 19, 22, 27, 49, 94]. Moreover, the specific nature of the V3 loop, based on whether it is from an R5 or X4 strain, is the primary determinant of direct Env chemokine receptor binding and Env-mediated inhibition of chemokine and monoclonal antibody binding to chemokine receptors [22, 105, 112].

3
Impact of Nonfunctional Chemokine Receptor Alleles on HIV-1 Resistance and Disease Progression

A mutation in the CCR5 open reading frame results in the premature truncation and a consequent 32-bp deletion in the protein (CCR5 Δ32). Although this mutation is relatively common in the Caucasian population, with an allele frequency of 15–20%, it was found to be significantly underrepresented in the HIV-1 infected groups [30, 88], and individuals homozygous for the mutation are only rarely infected with HIV [10, 45, 70, 77, 103]. In fact, in a group of people at high risk, two individuals that remained uninfected despite repeated exposure, were found to be homozygous for the same $\Delta ccr5$ mutation [60]. Lymphocytes from these individuals are resistant in vitro to M-tropic strains but permissive for T-tropic strains of HIV-1 [79]. In addition, HIV-1-infected individuals who are heterozygous for the $\Delta ccr5$ mutation have around a 2-year delay in their progression to AIDS compared to wildtype controls [30, 50, 69, 117]. These findings highlight the importance of CCR5 as a coreceptor in HIV-1 entry in humans.

In addition to the $\Delta ccr5$ mutation, other genetic polymorphisms have been found in certain chemokine receptors and their corresponding ligands. The CCR2-64I polymorphism causes a conservative valine to isoleucine mutation in CCR2. This mutation does not impact initial HIV transmission. However, individuals harboring this polymorphism progress to AIDS significantly slower (by 2–3 years) as compared to $CCR2^{+/+}$ HIV-1 seroconverters [55, 74, 84, 97]. Moreover, seropositive individuals who carry this allele in combination with the $\Delta ccr5$ allele experience an additive delay in the progression to symptomatic disease [55, 97]. The mechanism for this protective effect is not clear, as CCR2 does not appear to function as a coreceptor for HIV entry on primary cells, and CCR2-64I appears to have normal receptor function [57].

Another notable coreceptor polymorphism is the CCR5 59029 G/A single-nucleotide polymorphism. Both alleles, either G or A at position 59020 in the CCR5 promoter, are very common across racial groups. In one study, individuals selected for the absence of CCR5 $\Delta 32$ or CCR2-64I had a mean time to AIDS for 59029 G/G that was 3.8 years longer ($p=0.004$) than for 59029 A/A individuals [67]. In reporter gene assays, promoter fragments differing in sequence only at 59029 G versus A had differential activity, with the 59029 A promoter being more active than the 59029 G promoter [67], suggesting that 59029 G/G individuals might have decreased transcription and consequently lower expression of CCR5. This is consistent with the observation that CCR5 $\Delta 32$ heterozygotes progress to AIDS more slowly in the absence of therapy, strongly suggesting that CCR5 levels are rate-limiting for HIV infection in vivo.

The SDF-1 3'A allele is a G to A transition at position 809 of the 3'-untranslated region (UTR) of the messenger RNA (mRNA) encoding one of the two chemokine ligands for CXCR4, SDF-1β. In one report based on pooled seroconverters from three cohorts, a strong association was described between the 3'A/3'A genotype and delayed onset of AIDS [111]. However, in several subsequent reports, no association was found between homozygosity for the SDF-1 3'A allele and retarded progression to disease [13, 47, 66, 68, 74, 107].

Moreover, in an international meta-analysis study, the SDF-1 3′A allele was shown to not be predictive of disease outcome or progression [53].

Finally, individuals whose *CCL3L1* (*MIP1αP*) gene copy number is above the population median have a reduced risk for acquiring HIV with each stepwise increase in copy number of this gene [44]. Moreover, a gene dose lower than the overall cohort median or the population-specific median is associated with a dose-dependent increased risk of progressing rapidly to AIDS or death. Since CCL3L1 is a potent ligand for CCR5, it stands to reason that increasing CCL3L1 copy number leads to a reduction in the proportion of CD4-positive CCR5-expressing T cells and a consequent diminution in the risk of acquiring HIV as well as the rate of progression to AIDS.

4
Coreceptor-Based Antiretroviral Therapy

Since the discovery of chemokine receptors as coreceptors for HIV-1 entry, a significant focus of antiretroviral drug development has been directed toward antagonists of these receptors and their interactions with HIV-1 Env. The structures of some of the important coreceptor inhibitors discussed below are shown in Fig. 2. The HIV coreceptors are especially attractive drug targets, particularly CCR5, which is used by most primary HIV-1 strains. The strongest evidence for the importance of CCR5 in HIV-1 transmission and pathogenesis is the profound resistance to HIV-1 infection of individuals encoding two copies of a nonfunctional *ccr5* gene [60, 88]. The lack of serious immunological defects in humans homozygous for the inactivating 32-bp deletion (CCR5 Δ32) suggests that CCR5 may be a good therapeutic target.

4.1
CCR5-Based Antiretroviral Therapy

Early attempts at blocking CCR5 involved altered versions of the natural CCR5 ligands, MIP-1α, MIP-1β, and RANTES. These protein-based inhibitors blocked CCR5-mediated HIV-1 infection by competing with gp120 for the receptor-binding site, downregulation of receptor expression, and induction of receptor signaling events that altered cellular differentiation and susceptibility to HIV-1. Thus far, the poor pharmacokinetics and bioavailability of these drugs have prevented their development as candidates for antiretroviral therapeutics. However, the newer derivatives of RANTES (such as PSC-RANTES) might have potential as components of microbicides, as they can block vaginal transmission of virus in a rhesus macaque model [56].

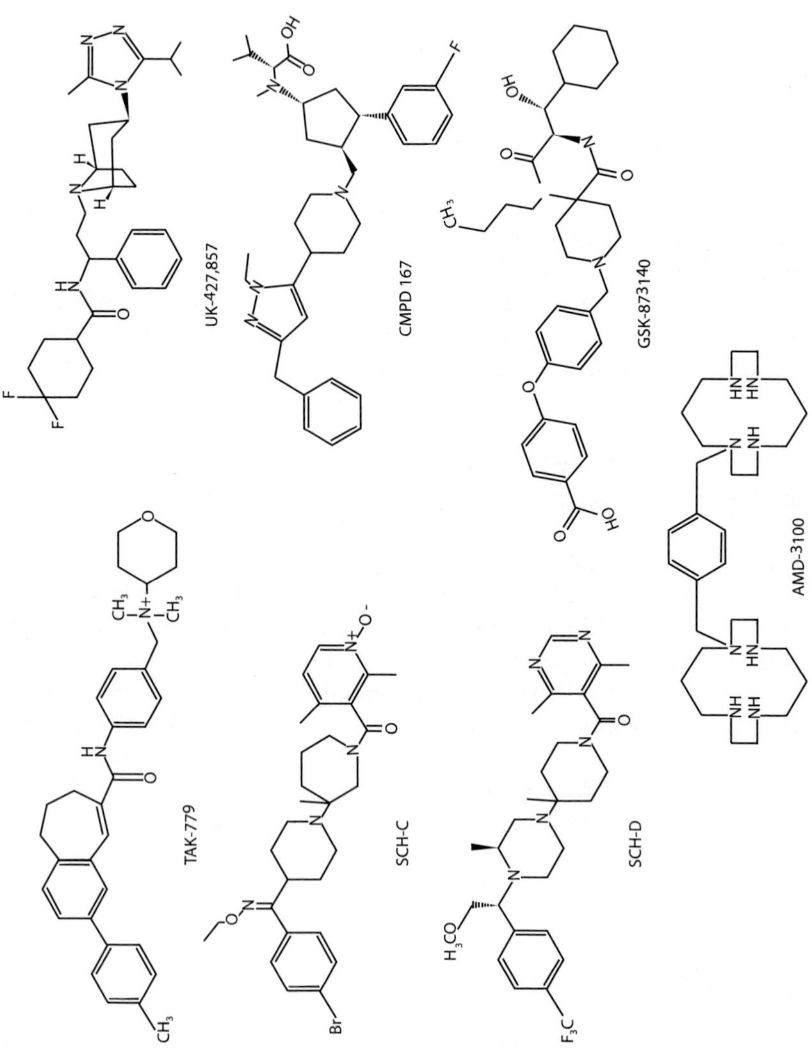

Fig. 2 Structures of CCR5 and CXCR4 inhibitors

4.1.1
TAK-779, TAK-220, and TAK-652

Small molecule inhibitors of CCR5 have proved to have significant potential as anti-HIV-1 therapy. TAK-779 was the first described small-molecule CCR5 inhibitor. This compound blocks CCR5-mediated signaling at nanomolar concentrations without any effects on CCR5 expression [6, 40]. Accordingly, the compound can block infection by R5- but not X4-tropic HIV-1 strains by interfering in the interaction between gp120 and CCR5. TAK-779 can also block binding to CCR2, which shares sequence homology with CCR5. Therefore, TAK-779 is able to block infection by simian immunodeficiency virus $(SIV)_{rcm}$, which uses CCR2 as its major coreceptor [113]. Despite its potent antiviral capacity, further development of TAK-779 was abandoned because it was not orally bioavailable and caused irritation at the site of injection [52].

However, a derivative of TAK-779, termed TAK-220, is orally bioavailable and is capable of blocking HIV-1 replication in PBMCs in the low nanomolar range. Specifically, TAK-220 can inhibit R5 HIV-1 isolates with IC_{50} and IC_{90} values of 1.1 nM and 13 nM [52, 104]. When administered orally to fasting rats and monkeys at a dose of 5 mg/kg, the bioavailability of TAK-220 was 9.5% and 28.9%, respectively [52]. TAK-220 also inhibits the binding of RANTES and MIP-1α to CCR5-expressing cells, but does not block binding of MIP-1β. Owing to its potent activity and favorable pharmacokinetics, TAK-220 is a candidate for clinical development.

Recently, another TAK-779 derivative, TAK-652, was described [5]. TAK-652 selectively inhibited R5 HIV-1 but not X4 HIV-1 replication. This compound was able to potently inhibit the replication of six R5 HIV-1 clinical isolates, including reverse transcriptase- and protease inhibitor-resistant mutants, with mean IC_{50} and IC_{90} values of 0.061 nM and 0.25 nM, respectively. In addition, all recombinant HIV-1 strains with seven different subtype (A to G) Env proteins were equally susceptible to TAK-652 with a mean IC_{50} of 1.0 nM. Single oral doses of TAK-652 (25–100 mg) were safe and well tolerated. TAK-652 showed good oral absorption, and its plasma concentration at 24 h after administration (25 mg) was 8.8 nM.

4.1.2
SCH-C and SCH-D

SCH-C is another small, non-peptide CCR5 antagonist that inhibits ligand binding to CCR5. SCH-C has broad and potent antiviral activity in vitro against primary R5-using HIV-1 isolates, with mean IC_{50} values between 0.4 and 9 nM [100]. High doses of SCH-C are also able to slightly inhibit ligand binding to CCR2. SCH-C can strongly inhibit replication of an R5-using HIV-1 isolate in vivo in severe combined immunodeficiency (SCID)-hu Thy/Liv mice [100]. The compound has also shown favorable pharmacokinetics in rodents and primates, with an oral bioavailability of 50%–60% and a serum half-life of 5–6 h. Clinical data obtained from an early human trial where SCH-C monotherapy was administered (25 mg twice daily) to HIV-infected adults for 10 days demonstrated viral load reductions between 0.5 and 1.0 $\log_{10}$ [83]. However the same study found a prolongation of the QT_c interval, suggesting possible adverse cardiac effects at high doses, resulting in cessation of further development of this compound.

SCH-D, a derivative of SCH-C, was shown to have greater potency in vitro and in vivo [92]. In a phase I clinical trial, SCH-D monotherapy with escalating doses of 10–50 mg twice daily over 14 days, no adverse effects were seen. A dose-dependent reduction in plasma viremia was observed, with mean reductions of up to 1.62 $\log_{10}$ [92].

4.1.3
UK-427857 (Maraviroc)

Another CCR5 inhibitor, UK-427857 (recently termed maraviroc), potently blocks cell entry of a range of lab-adapted and primary R5-tropic HIV-1 isolates in vitro (IC_{90}<10 nM) [38]. Despite its potency against R5-tropic isolates, the compound is specific and remains inactive against X4-tropic isolates [38]. UK-427857 blocks gp120 and chemokine ligand binding to CCR5, but does not induce intracellular signaling or trigger receptor internalization [38]. UK-427857 is orally bioavailable, has favorable pharmacokinetics, and did not have any serious adverse effects on healthy volunteers [2]. In a study evaluating the effects of short-term (10 days) UK-427857 monotherapy on HIV viral load in HIV patients, subjects received 25 mg of the drug once a day, 100 mg twice daily, or a placebo for 10 days. The mean CCR5 receptor saturation at the 100-mg dose was in excess of 90% and the mean decrease in viral load was 1.42 $\log_{10}$ from baseline to day 11 [80]. At the 25-mg dose, the mean receptor saturation fell to less than 80% by day 10 and the mean decrease in viral load was 0.42 $\log_{10}$ [80]. The absence of any severe adverse effects combined with the potent antiviral properties of UK-427857 make it an attractive candidate for further development.

4.1.4
CMPD 167

CMPD 167 is a cyclopentane-based compound that can cause rapid and significant decline in plasma viremia in rhesus macaques chronically infected with SIV [108]. Moreover, vaginal application of gel-formulated CMPD 167 prevented vaginal SIV transmission in 2 out of 11 animals, and reduced early viral replication in all 11 animals receiving the drug compared to control-treated animals. These results provide a proof of principle for the use of small-molecule CCR5 inhibitors as a component of a topical microbicide to prevent HIV-1 sexual transmission. However, CMPD 167 is no longer being developed as an anti-HIV-1 therapeutic agent.

4.1.5
Spirodiketopiperazine-Based Inhibitors

The first spirodiketopiperazine (SDP) derivative, E913, was described in 2001. E913 was active against R5-tropic HIV-1 in vitro, with IC_{50} values of 30–60 nM in PBMCs [64]. Subsequently, a more potent SDP derivative, AK602/GSK-873140, was described [31, 62]. In vitro, AK602 had potent antiviral activity against a wide range of laboratory and primary R5 HIV-1 isolates, including multidrug-resistant strains, with IC_{50} values ranging from 0.1 to 0.6 nM. The variability of this antiviral activity was low (similar to zidovudine), probably owing to the high potency of AK602 as compared with E913 or TAK-779. AK602 binds with high affinity to CCR5 (K_d=2.9±1.0) and specifically blocks binding of MIP-1α even though it preserves RANTES and MIP-1β binding and their functions, including CC chemokine-induced chemotaxis and CCR5 internalization. In a nonobese diabetic SCID mouse model, AK602 elicited a 2.0 $\log_{10}$ decline in plasma viremia in R5 HIV_{JRFL}-infected mice [63]. In a phase I clinical trial involving multiple-dose escalation in healthy subjects, AK602 was well tolerated and had no severe adverse effects. A phase II clinical trial of AK602 is currently underway.

4.2
CXCR4-Based Antiretroviral Therapy

As mentioned earlier, CXCR4 is the other major coreceptor commonly involved in HIV-1 infection in vivo [43]. CXCR4 is expressed on most CD4-positive lymphocytes as well as on many cell types that lack CD4 [58]. In some but not all individuals who progress to AIDS, viruses evolve to use CXCR4 for entry either in addition to or in place of CCR5 [25]. While this coreceptor switch is not required for disease progression, it does result in expanded viral tropism, since CXCR4 is more commonly expressed on CD4-positive T cells than is CCR5 [12].

4.2.1
Small Molecule CXCR4 Inhibitors

Inhibitors of CXCR4 are also under development, but these drugs may be more difficult to field because CXCR4, and its ligand SDF-1α, are essential for normal development in the mouse [118]. AMD-3100 is a bicyclam compound that disrupts the interaction of gp120 and CXCR4 and is capable of blocking replication of CXCR4 utilizing strains in vitro and in murine models [34, 48, 90]. AMD-3100 is very specific for CXCR4 and does not interact with any other known CXC- or CC-chemokine receptor [26]. An orally bioavailable AMD-3100 derivative, AMD-070, is currently in clinical trials. Several other CXCR4 antagonists have been described including polyphemusin analogs T22, T134, and T140, as well as a D-Arg peptide referred to as ALX40-4C [36, 75]. ALX40-4C was well tolerated in a phase I clinical trial, suggesting but not proving that CXCR4 inhibition may be tolerated in adults [35].

5
Resistance to Coreceptor Inhibitors

HIV-1 can acquire resistance to coreceptor inhibitors either by changing the mechanism or dynamics of coreceptor engagement or by switching coreceptor usage. The former could involve usage of the same coreceptor in a drug-bound form, increased affinity of the virus for the coreceptor leading to competitive removal of bound inhibitor molecules, or easier triggering of Env trimers resulting in membrane fusion even at low coreceptor density. For R5-tropic viruses, in particular, coreceptor switching (from R5 to X4) is a matter of concern because the presence of X4-tropic viruses is associated with advanced stages of disease and poor prognosis. Many of the studies addressing selection of viruses resistant to coreceptor inhibitors have used cell lines that express only one coreceptor [1, 29, 54, 65, 89]. Consequently, the resistant viruses selected in these studies did not have display coreceptor switching, but rather had alterations in how the virus bound to the original coreceptor.

In cells expressing both CCR5 and CXCR4, coreceptor switching of viruses passaged in the presence of coreceptor antagonists has been observed [73, 106]. For instance, when an R5 virus was passaged in the presence of AD101 (a CCR5 antagonist), the virus evolved to use CCR5 via an inhibitor-independent mechanism [106]. Similar results were observed with SCH-C, another CCR5 inhibitor [72, 106]. Finally, when X4 and R5X4-tropic viruses were passaged in the presence of the CXCR4 antagonist AMD-3100, R5 viruses expanded in the cultures [41, 46]. When CCR5 viruses persisted in the presence of AD101, the selected variants had various amino acid changes in Env, did not use CXCR4 for entry, and were able to replicate efficiently in PBMCs in a CCR5-dependent manner [106]. Despite their newly acquired resistance, these variants used CCR5 with reduced efficiency for entry into cell lines, implying that resistance might be associated with a loss in viral fitness [106].

Another possible mechanism by which HIV-1 could evolve resistance to CCR5 or CXCR4 inhibitors would be to acquire the ability to use alternative coreceptors for virus entry. Switching to alternative coreceptors has not yet been observed. However, in an experimental setting where CCR5-negative peripheral blood lymphocytes (PBLs) were infected with an R5/X4/CXCR6-tropic HIV-1 isolate in the presence of AMD-3100, CXCR6-positive PBLs were preferentially infected [93]. This suggests that CXCR6 can be used as a coreceptor by HIV-1 on primary cells, and further that in the presence of CCR5 and CXCR4 inhibitors, variants using CXCR6 (or other minor coreceptor) might arise in vivo in tissues that express high amounts of minor coreceptors. It is also worth noting that SIV strains isolated from red-capped mangabeys often use CCR2 as their major coreceptor, perhaps because many red-capped mangabeys are CCR5-negative due to a naturally occurring polymorphism in the CCR5 open reading frame [16]. This represents an example of novel coreceptor use in the face of strong selective pressure. Theoretically, this could also occur in humans, though based on the expression patterns and levels of alternative coreceptors in humans we feel that resistance to CCR5 inhibitors in humans will likely involve either altered use of CCR5 by virus, or by coreceptor switching to CXCR4.

6
Impact of Chemokine Receptor Inhibitors on Clinical Monitoring and Treatment

Accurate and timely clinical monitoring is an integral part of any effective antiretroviral therapeutic regimen. Viral genotyping to determine specific resistance-associated mutations is increasingly becoming part of the clinical monitoring process. In the context of coreceptor antagonists, it will be particularly important to assess the relative proportions of R5, R5X4, and X4 viruses in individuals prior to initiating treatment. CCR5 inhibitors may not be beneficial to patients with X4 viruses and vice versa for CXCR4 inhibitors. Moreover, the possibility of coreceptor switching (from R5 to X4) will have to be carefully monitored. Monitoring host factors that might impact CCR5 expression could also prove useful in predicting treatment success, since CCR5 levels can influence the efficacy of coreceptor antagonists [81]. At present, phenotyping tests on cell lines expressing CCR5 or CXCR4 along with CD4 are used to measure the relative levels of coreceptor use on patient samples. However, it is not clear how results from these in vitro tests translate to coreceptor use in vivo.

As various entry inhibitors move through clinical development, it will be important to determine if particular combinations of entry inhibitors should be used. Coreceptor inhibitors effectively reduce the levels of coreceptor available to virus. As a result, virus entry is either inhibited or the rate of virus entry is slowed. As a consequence of slower fusion rates, virus becomes more susceptible to the fusion inhibitor T-20 (enfuvirtide) [81]. Enfuvirtide binds to a region on gp41 that becomes exposed as a result of CD4 binding, but that is lost once coreceptor binding triggers membrane fusion [15]. Slower coreceptor binding causes the T-20 binding site to be exposed for a longer period of time, resulting in synergistic inhibition of virus fusion [81, 82]. This finding provides a strong theoretical basis for using coreceptor inhibitors in conjunction with T-20. Moreover, since T-20 can inhibit both R5- and X4-tropic viruses, the use of T-20 in conjunction with a CCR5 inhibitor may limit the evolution of X4-tropic virus strains.

It is also possible that particular combinations of coreceptor inhibitors could be used together effectively, much like nucleoside and nonnucleoside reverse transcriptase inhibitors that are used in combination. In fact, a recent study reported greater synergism of the CCR5 inhibitor AK602/GSK-873140 with CXCR4 inhibitors (such as AMD-3100) than with other classes of anti-HIV drugs [76]. Another recent study indicates that virus resistance to some CCR5 inhibitors may not result in resistance to other CCR5 inhibitors. Specifically, a virus resistant to UK-427857 remained sensitive to CCR5 inhibitors with a different structure [109]. As a result, it may be possible to apply different classes of CCR5 inhibitors in combination—or sequentially—should resistance to one inhibitor arise. In conclusion, coreceptor antagonists constitute an important and valuable new class of drugs, and with careful monitoring and synergistic use, they can be successfully incorporated into an efficacious antiretroviral regimen.

References

1. Aarons E, Beddows S, Willingham T, Wu L, Koup R (2001) Adaptation to blockade of human immunodeficiency virus type 1 entry imposed by the anti-CCR5 monoclonal antibody 2D7. Virology 287:382–390
2. Abel S, Van der Ryst E, Muirhead GJ, Rosario M, Edgington A, Weissgerber G (2003) Pharmacokinetics of single and multiple oral doses of UK-427,857—a novel CCR5 antagonist in healthy volunteers [abstr]. Program and abstracts of the 10th Conference on Retroviruses and Opportunistic Infections, 10–14 February 2003. Abstr 556
3. Alkhatib G, Combadiere C, Broder CC, Feng Y, Kennedy PE, Murphy PM, Berger EA (1996) CC CKR5: a RANTES, MIP-1alpha, MIP-1beta receptor as a fusion cofactor for macrophage-tropic HIV-1. Science 272:1955–1958
4. Ashorn PA, Berger EA, Moss B (1990) Human immunodeficiency virus envelope glycoprotein/CD4-mediated fusion of nonprimate cells with human cells. J Virol 64:2149–2156

5. Baba M, Kanzaki N, Miyake H, Wang X, Takashima K, Teshima K, Shiraishi M, Iizawa Y (2005) TAK-652, a novel small molecule CCR5 antagonist with potent anti-HIV-1 activity. Program and abstracts of the 12th Conference on Retroviruses and Opportunistic Infections, 22–25 February 2005, Boston. Abstr 541
6. Baba M, Nishimura O, Kanzaki N, Okamoto M, Sawada H, Iizawa Y, Shiraishi M, Aramaki Y, Okonogi K, Ogawa Y, Meguro K, Fujino M (1999) A small-molecule, nonpeptide CCR5 antagonist with highly potent and selective anti-HIV-1 activity. Proc Natl Acad Sci USA 96:5698–5703
7. Bazan HA, Alkhatib G, Broder CC, Berger EA (1998) Patterns of CCR5, CXCR4, and CCR3 usage by envelope glycoproteins from human immunodeficiency virus type 1 primary isolates. J Virol 72:4485–4491
8. Berger EA, Murphy PM, Farber JM (1999) Chemokine receptors as HIV-1 coreceptors: roles in viral entry, tropism, and disease. Annu Rev Immunol 17:657–700
9. Bieniasz PD, Fridell RA, Aramori I, Ferguson SS, Caron MG, Cullen BR (1997) HIV-1-induced cell fusion is mediated by multiple regions within both the viral envelope and the CCR-5 co-receptor. EMBO J 16:2599–2609
10. Biti R, Ffrench R, Young J, Bennetts B, Stewart G, Liang T (1997) HIV-1 infection in an individual homozygous for the CCR5 deletion allele. Nat Med 3:252–253
11. Bleul CC, Farzan M, Choe H, Parolin C, Clark-Lewis I, Sodroski J, Springer TA (1996) The lymphocyte chemoattractant SDF-1 is a ligand for LESTR/fusin and blocks HIV-1 entry. Nature 382:829–833
12. Bleul CC, Wu L, Hoxie JA, Springer TA, Mackay CR (1997) The HIV coreceptors CXCR4 and CCR5 are differentially expressed and regulated on human T lymphocytes. Proc Natl Acad Sci USA 94:1925–1930
13. Brambilla A, Villa C, Rizzardi G, Veglia F, Ghezzi S, Lazzarin A, Cusini M, Muratori S, Santagostino E, Gringeri A, Louie LG, Sheppard HW, Poli G, Michael NL, Pantaleo G, Vicenzi E (2000) Shorter survival of SDF1-3'A/3'A homozygotes linked to CD4+ T cell decrease in advanced human immunodeficiency virus type 1 infection. J Infect Dis 182:311–315
14. Broder CC, Dimitrov DS, Blumenthal R, Berger EA (1993) The block to HIV-1 envelope glycoprotein-mediated membrane fusion in animal cells expressing human CD4 can be overcome by a human cell component(s). Virology 193:483–491
15. Chen CH, Matthews TJ, McDanal CB, Bolognesi DP, Greenberg ML (1995) A molecular clasp in the human immunodeficiency virus (HIV) type 1 TM protein determines the anti-HIV activity of gp41 derivatives: implication for viral fusion. J Virol 69:3771–3777
16. Chen Z, Kwon D, Jin Z, Monard S, Telfer P, Jones MS, Lu CY, Aguilar RF, Ho DD, Marx PA (1998) Natural infection of a homozygous delta24 CCR5 red-capped mangabey with an R2b-tropic simian immunodeficiency virus. J Exp Med 188:2057–2065
17. Chesebro B, Nishio J, Perryman S, Cann A, O'Brien W, Chen IS, Wehrly K (1991) Identification of human immunodeficiency virus envelope gene sequences influencing viral entry into CD4-positive HeLa cells, T-leukemia cells, and macrophages. J Virol 65:5782–5789

18. Chesebro B, Wehrly K, Nishio J, Perryman S (1992) Macrophage-tropic human immunodeficiency virus isolates from different patients exhibit unusual V3 envelope sequence homogeneity in comparison with T-cell-tropic isolates: definition of critical amino acids involved in cell tropism. J Virol 66:6547–6554
19. Choe H, Farzan M, Sun Y, Sullivan N, Rollins B, Ponath PD, Wu L, Mackay CR, LaRosa G, Newman W, Gerard N, Gerard C, Sodroski J (1996) The beta-chemokine receptors CCR3 and CCR5 facilitate infection by primary HIV-1 isolates. Cell 85:1135–1148
20. Clapham PR, Blanc D, Weiss RA (1991) Specific cell surface requirements for the infection of CD4-positive cells by human immunodeficiency virus types 1 and 2 and by Simian immunodeficiency virus. Virology 181:703–715
21. Cocchi F, DeVico AL, Garzino-Demo A, Arya SK, Gallo RC, Lusso P (1995) Identification of RANTES, MIP-1 alpha, and MIP-1 beta as the major HIV-suppressive factors produced by CD8+ T cells. Science 270:1811–1815
22. Cocchi F, DeVico AL, Garzino-Demo A, Cara A, Gallo RC, Lusso P (1996) The V3 domain of the HIV-1 gp120 envelope glycoprotein is critical for chemokine-mediated blockade of infection. Nat Med 2:1244–1247
23. Connor RI, Mohri H, Cao Y, Ho DD (1993) Increased viral burden and cytopathicity correlate temporally with CD4+ T-lymphocyte decline and clinical progression in human immunodeficiency virus type 1-infected individuals. J Virol 67:1772–1777
24. [Reference deleted in proof]
25. Connor RI, Sheridan KE, Ceradini D, Choe S, Landau NR (1997) Change in coreceptor use coreceptor use correlates with disease progression in HIV-1-infected individuals. J Exp Med 185:621–628
26. De Clercq E (2003) The bicyclam AMD3100 story. Nat Rev Drug Discov 2:581–587
27. De Jong JJ, De Ronde A, Keulen W, Tersmette M, Goudsmit J (1992) Minimal requirements for the human immunodeficiency virus type 1 V3 domain to support the syncytium-inducing phenotype: analysis by single amino acid substitution. J Virol 66:6777–6780
28. de Jong JJ, Goudsmit J, Keulen W, Klaver B, Krone W, Tersmette M, de Ronde A (1992) Human immunodeficiency virus type 1 clones chimeric for the envelope V3 domain differ in syncytium formation and replication capacity. J Virol 66:757–765
29. de Vreese K, Kofler-Mongold V, Leutgeb C, Weber V, Vermeire K, Schacht S, Anne J, de Clercq E, Datema R, Werner G (1996) The molecular target of bicyclams, potent inhibitors of human immunodeficiency virus replication. J Virol 70:689–696
30. Dean M, Carrington M, Winkler C, Huttley GA, Smith MW, Allikmets R, Goedert JJ, Buchbinder SP, Vittinghoff E, Gomperts E, Donfield S, Vlahov D, Kaslow R, Saah A, Rinaldo C, Detels R, O'Brien SJ (1996) Genetic restriction of HIV-1 infection and progression to AIDS by a deletion allele of the CKR5 structural gene. Hemophilia Growth and Development Study, Multicenter AIDS Cohort Study, Multicenter Hemophilia Cohort Study, San Francisco City Cohort, ALIVE Study. Science 273:1856–1862

31. Demarest J, Adkison K, Sparks S, Shachoy-Clark A, Schell K, Reddy S, Fang L, O'-Mara K, Shibayama S, Piscitelli S (2004) Single and multiple dose escalation study to investigate the safety, pharmacokinetics, and receptor binding of GW873140, a novel CCR5 receptor antagonist in healthy subjects. Program and abstracts of the 11th Conference on Retroviruses and Opportunistic Infections, 8–11 February 2004, San Francisco. Abstr 139
32. Deng H, Liu R, Ellmeier W, Choe S, Unutmaz D, Burkhart M, Di Marzio P, Marmon S, Sutton RE, Hill CM, Davis CB, Peiper SC, Schall TJ, Littman DR, Landau NR (1996) Identification of a major co-receptor for primary isolates of HIV-1. Nature 381:661–666
33. Deng HK, Unutmaz D, KewalRamani VN, Littman DR (1997) Expression cloning of new receptors used by simian and human immunodeficiency viruses. Nature 388:296–300
34. Donzella GA, Schols D, Lin SW, Este JA, Nagashima KA, Maddon PJ, Allaway GP, Sakmar TP, Henson G, De Clercq E, Moore JP (1998) AMD3100, a small molecule inhibitor of HIV-1 entry via the CXCR4 co-receptor. Nat Med 4:72–77
35. Doranz BJ, Filion LG, Diaz-Mitoma F, Sitar DS, Sahai J, Baribaud F, Orsini MJ, Benovic JL, Cameron W, Doms RW (2001) Safe use of the CXCR4 inhibitor ALX40-4C in humans. AIDS Res Hum Retroviruses 17:475–486
36. Doranz BJ, Grovit-Ferbas K, Sharron MP, Mao SH, Goetz MB, Daar ES, Doms RW, O'Brien WA (1997) A small-molecule inhibitor directed against the chemokine receptor CXCR4 prevents its use as an HIV-1 coreceptor. J Exp Med 186:1395–1400
37. Doranz BJ, Rucker J, Yi Y, Smyth RJ, Samson M, Peiper SC, Parmentier M, Collman RG, Doms RW (1996) A dual-tropic primary HIV-1 isolate that uses fusin and the beta-chemokine receptors CKR-5, CKR-3, and CKR-2b as fusion cofactors. Cell 85:1149–1158
38. Dorr P, Macartney M, Rickett G, Smith-Burchnell C, Dobbs S, Mori J, Griffin P, Lok J, Irvine R, Westby M, Hitchcock C, Stammen B, et al (2003) UK-427,857, a novel small molecule HIV entry inhibitor is a specific antagonist of the chemokine receptor CCR5. Program and abstracts of the 10th Conference on Retroviruses and Opportunistic Infections, 10–14 February 2003, Boston. Abstr 12
39. Dragic T, Litwin V, Allaway GP, Martin SR, Huang Y, Nagashima KA, Cayanan C, Maddon PJ, Koup RA, Moore JP, Paxton WA (1996) HIV-1 entry into CD4+ cells is mediated by the chemokine receptor CC-CKR-5. Nature 381:667–673
40. Dragic T, Trkola A, Thompson DA, Cormier EG, Kajumo FA, Maxwell E, Lin SW, Ying W, Smith SO, Sakmar TP, Moore JP (2000) A binding pocket for a small molecule inhibitor of HIV-1 entry within the transmembrane helices of CCR5. Proc Natl Acad Sci U S A 97:5639–5644
41. Este JA, Cabrera C, Blanco J, Gutierrez A, Bridger G, Henson G, Clotet B, Schols D, De Clercq E (1999) Shift of clinical human immunodeficiency virus type 1 isolates from X4 to R5 and prevention of emergence of the syncytium-inducing phenotype by blockade of CXCR4. J Virol 73:5577–5585
42. [Reference deleted in proof]
43. Feng Y, Broder CC, Kennedy PE, Berger EA (1996) HIV-1 entry cofactor: functional cDNA cloning of a seven-transmembrane, G protein-coupled receptor. Science 272:872–877

44. Gonzalez E, Kulkarni H, Bolivar H, Mangano A, Sanchez R, Catano G, Nibbs RJ, Freedman BI, Quinones MP, Bamshad MJ, Murthy KK, Rovin BH, Bradley W, Clark RA, Anderson SA, O'Connell R J, Agan BK, Ahuja SS, Bologna R, Sen L, Dolan MJ, Ahuja SK (2005) The influence of CCL3L1 gene-containing segmental duplications on HIV-1/AIDS susceptibility. Science 307:1434–1440
45. Gorry PR, Zhang C, Wu S, Kunstman K, Trachtenberg E, Phair J, Wolinsky S, Gabuzda D (2002) Persistence of dual-tropic HIV-1 in an individual homozygous for the CCR5 Delta 32 allele. Lancet 359:1832–1834
46. Gotoh K, Yoshimori M, Kanbara K, Tamamura H, Kanamoto T, Mochizuki K, Fujii N, Nakashima H (2001) Increase of R5 HIV-1 infection and CCR5 expression in T cells treated with high concentrations of CXCR4 antagonists and SDF-1. J Infect Chemother 7:28–36
47. Hendel H, Henon N, Lebuanec H, Lachgar A, Poncelet H, Caillat-Zucman S, Winkler CA, Smith MW, Kenefic L, O'Brien S, Lu W, Andrieu JM, Zagury D, Schachter F, Rappaport J, Zagury JF (1998) Distinctive effects of CCR5, CCR2, and SDF1 genetic polymorphisms in AIDS progression. J Acquir Immune Defic Syndr Hum Retrovirol 19:381–386
48. Hendrix C, Collier AC, Lederman M, Pollard R, Brown S, Glesby M, et al (2002) Calandra for the AMD-3100 HIV Study Group. AMD-3100 CXCR4 receptor blocker fails to reduce HIV viral load by > 1 log following 10-day continuous infusion. 9th Conference on Retroviruses and Opportunistic Infections, Seattle. Abstr 391
49. Hoffman TL, Stephens EB, Narayan O, Doms RW (1998) HIV type I envelope determinants for use of the CCR2b, CCR3, STRL33, and APJ coreceptors. Proc Natl Acad Sci U S A 95:11360–11365
50. Huang Y, Paxton WA, Wolinsky SM, Neumann AU, Zhang L, He T, Kang S, Ceradini D, Jin Z, Yazdanbakhsh K, Kunstman K, Erickson D, Dragon E, Landau NR, Phair J, Ho DD, Koup RA (1996) The role of a mutant CCR5 allele in HIV-1 transmission and disease progression. Nat Med 2:1240–1243
51. Hwang SS, Boyle TJ, Lyerly HK, Cullen BR (1991) Identification of the envelope V3 loop as the primary determinant of cell tropism in HIV-1. Science 253:71–74
52. Iizawa Y, Kanzaki N, Takashima K, Miyake H, Tagawa Y, Sugihara Y, Baba M (2003) Anti-HIV-1 activity of TAK-220, a small molecule CCR5 antagonist. Program and abstracts of the 10th Conference on Retroviruses and Opportunistic Infections, 10–14 February 2003, Boston. Abstr 11
53. Ioannidis JP, Rosenberg PS, Goedert JJ, Ashton LJ, Benfield TL, Buchbinder SP, Coutinho RA, Eugen-Olsen J, Gallart T, Katzenstein TL, Kostrikis LG, Kuipers H, Louie LG, Mallal SA, Margolick JB, Martinez OP, Meyer L, Michael NL, Operskalski E, Pantaleo G, Rizzardi GP, Schuitemaker H, Sheppard HW, Stewart GJ, Theodorou ID, Ullum H, Vicenzi E, Vlahov D, Wilkinson D, Workman C, Zagury JF, O'Brien TR (2001) Effects of CCR5-Delta32, CCR2-64I, and SDF-1 3'A alleles on HIV-1 disease progression: An international meta-analysis of individual-patient data. Ann Intern Med 135:782–795
54. Kanbara K, Sato S, Tanuma J, Tamamura H, Gotoh K, Yoshimori M, Kanamoto T, Kitano M, Fujii N, Nakashima H (2001) Biological and genetic characterization of a human immunodeficiency virus strain resistant to CXCR4 antagonist T134. AIDS Res Hum Retroviruses 17:615–622

55. Kostrikis LG, Huang Y, Moore JP, Wolinsky SM, Zhang L, Guo Y, Deutsch L, Phair J, Neumann AU, Ho DD (1998) A chemokine receptor CCR2 allele delays HIV-1 disease progression and is associated with a CCR5 promoter mutation. Nat Med 4:350–353
56. Lederman MM, Veazey RS, Offord R, Mosier DE, Dufour J, Mefford M, Piatak M Jr, Lifson JD, Salkowitz JR, Rodriguez B, Blauvelt A, Hartley O (2004) Prevention of vaginal SHIV transmission in rhesus macaques through inhibition of CCR5. Science 306:485–487
57. Lee B, Doranz BJ, Rana S, Yi Y, Mellado M, Frade JM, Martinez AC, O'Brien SJ, Dean M, Collman RG, Doms RW (1998) Influence of the CCR2-V64I polymorphism on human immunodeficiency virus type 1 coreceptor activity and on chemokine receptor function of CCR2b, CCR3, CCR5, and CXCR4. J Virol 72:7450–7458
58. Lee B, Sharron M, Montaner LJ, Weissman D, Doms RW (1999) Quantification of CD4, CCR5, and CXCR4 levels on lymphocyte subsets, dendritic cells, and differentially conditioned monocyte-derived macrophages. Proc Natl Acad Sci USA 96:5215–5220
59. [Reference deleted in proof]
60. Liu R, Paxton WA, Choe S, Ceradini D, Martin SR, Horuk R, MacDonald ME, Stuhlmann H, Koup RA, Landau NR (1996) Homozygous defect in HIV-1 coreceptor accounts for resistance of some multiply-exposed individuals to HIV-1 infection. Cell 86:367–377
61. Maddon PJ, Dalgleish AG, McDougal JS, Clapham PR, Weiss RA, Axel R (1986) The T4 gene encodes the AIDS virus receptor and is expressed in the immune system and the brain. Cell 47:333–348
62. Maeda K, Nakata H, Koh Y, Miyakawa T, Ogata H, Takaoka Y, Shibayama S, Sagawa K, Fukushima D, Moravek J, Koyanagi Y, Mitsuya H (2004) Spirodiketopiperazine-based CCR5 inhibitor which preserves CC-chemokine/CCR5 interactions and exerts potent activity against R5 human immunodeficiency virus type 1 in vitro. J Virol 78:8654–8662
63. Maeda K, Nakata H, Ogata H, Koh Y, Miyakawa T, Mitsuya H (2004) The current status of, and challenges in, the development of CCR5 inhibitors as therapeutics for HIV-1 infection. Curr Opin Pharmacol 4:447–452
64. Maeda K, Yoshimura K, Shibayama S, Habashita H, Tada H, Sagawa K, Miyakawa T, Aoki M, Fukushima D, Mitsuya H (2001) Novel low molecular weight spirodiketopiperazine derivatives potently inhibit R5 HIV-1 infection through their antagonistic effects on CCR5. J Biol Chem 276:35194–35200
65. Maeda Y, Foda M, Matsushita S, Harada S (2000) Involvement of both the V2 and V3 regions of the CCR5-tropic human immunodeficiency virus type 1 envelope in reduced sensitivity to macrophage inflammatory protein 1alpha. J Virol 74:1787–1793
66. Magierowska M, Theodorou I, Debre P, Sanson F, Autran B, Riviere Y, Charron D, Costagliola D (1999) Combined genotypes of CCR5, CCR2, SDF1, and HLA genes can predict the long-term nonprogressor status in human immunodeficiency virus-1-infected individuals. Blood 93:936–941

67. McDermott DH, Zimmerman PA, Guignard F, Kleeberger CA, Leitman SF, Murphy PM (1998) CCR5 promoter polymorphism and HIV-1 disease progression. Multicenter AIDS Cohort Study (MACS). Lancet 352:866–870
68. Meyer L, Magierowska M, Hubert JB, Theodorou I, van Rij R, Prins M, de Roda Husman AM, Coutinho R, Schuitemaker H (1999) CC-chemokine receptor variants, SDF-1 polymorphism, and disease progression in 720 HIV-infected patients. SEROCO Cohort. Amsterdam Cohort Studies on AIDS. Aids 13:624–626
69. Michael NL, Chang G, Louie LG, Mascola JR, Dondero D, Birx DL, Sheppard HW (1997) The role of viral phenotype and CCR-5 gene defects in HIV-1 transmission and disease progression. Nat Med 3:338–340
70. Michael NL, Nelson JA, KewalRamani VN, Chang G, O'Brien SJ, Mascola JR, Volsky B, Louder M, White GC 2nd, Littman DR, Swanstrom R, O'Brien TR (1998) Exclusive and persistent use of the entry coreceptor CXCR4 by human immunodeficiency virus type 1 from a subject homozygous for CCR5 delta32. J Virol 72:6040–6047
71. Miedema F, Meyaard L, Koot M, Klein MR, Roos MT, Groenink M, Fouchier RA, Van't Wout AB, Tersmette M, Schellekens PT, et al (1994) Changing virus-host interactions in the course of HIV-1 infection. Immunol Rev 140:35–72
72. Moore JP, Doms RW (2003) The entry of entry inhibitors: a fusion of science and medicine. Proc Natl Acad Sci U S A 100:10598–10602
73. Mosier DE, Picchio GR, Gulizia RJ, Sabbe R, Poignard P, Picard L, Offord RE, Thompson DA, Wilken J (1999) Highly potent RANTES analogues either prevent CCR5-using human immunodeficiency virus type 1 infection in vivo or rapidly select for CXCR4-using variants. J Virol 73:3544–3550
74. Mummidi S, Ahuja SS, Gonzalez E, Anderson SA, Santiago EN, Stephan KT, Craig FE, O'Connell P, Tryon V, Clark RA, Dolan MJ, Ahuja SK (1998) Genealogy of the CCR5 locus and chemokine system gene variants associated with altered rates of HIV-1 disease progression. Nat Med 4:786–793
75. Murakami T, Nakajima T, Koyanagi Y, Tachibana K, Fujii N, Tamamura H, Yoshida N, Waki M, Matsumoto A, Yoshie O, Kishimoto T, Yamamoto N, Nagasawa T (1997) A small molecule CXCR4 inhibitor that blocks T cell line-tropic HIV-1 infection. J Exp Med 186:1389–1393
76. Nakata H, Koh Y, Maeda K, Takaoka Y, Tamamura H, Fujii N, Mitsuya H (2005) Greater synergistic anti-HIV effects upon combinations of a CCR5 inhibitor AK602/ONO4128/GW873140 with CXCR4 inhibitors than with other anti-HIV drugs. Program and abstracts of the 12th Conference on Retroviruses and Opportunistic Infections, 22–25 February 2005, Boston. Abstr 543
77. O'Brien TR, Winkler C, Dean M, Nelson JA, Carrington M, Michael NL, White GC 2nd (1997) HIV-1 infection in a man homozygous for CCR5 delta 32. Lancet 349:1219
78. Oberlin E, Amara A, Bachelerie F, Bessia C, Virelizier JL, Arenzana-Seisdedos F, Schwartz O, Heard JM, Clark-Lewis I, Legler DF, Loetscher M, Baggiolini M, Moser B (1996) The CXC chemokine SDF-1 is the ligand for LESTR/fusin and prevents infection by T-cell-line-adapted HIV-1. Nature 382:833–835

79. Paxton WA, Martin SR, Tse D, O'Brien TR, Skurnick J, VanDevanter NL, Padian N, Braun JF, Kotler DP, Wolinsky SM, Koup RA (1996) Relative resistance to HIV-1 infection of CD4 lymphocytes from persons who remain uninfected despite multiple high-risk sexual exposure. Nat Med 2:412–417
80. Pozniak AL, Fatkenheuer G, Johnson M, Hoepelman IM, Rockstroh J, Goebel F, Abel S, James I, Rosario M, Medhurst C, et al (2003) Presented at the 43rd Annual Interscience Conference on Antimicrobial Agents and Chemotherapy, Chicago. Abstr H-443
81. Reeves JD, Gallo SA, Ahmad N, Miamidian JL, Harvey PE, Sharron M, Pohlmann S, Sfakianos JN, Derdeyn CA, Blumenthal R, Hunter E, Doms RW (2002) Sensitivity of HIV-1 to entry inhibitors correlates with envelope/coreceptor affinity, receptor density, and fusion kinetics. Proc Natl Acad Sci USA 99:16249–16254
82. Reeves JD, Miamidian JL, Biscone MJ, Lee FH, Ahmad N, Pierson TC, Doms RW (2004) Impact of mutations in the coreceptor binding site on human immunodeficiency virus type 1 fusion, infection, and entry inhibitor sensitivity. J Virol 78:5476–5485
83. Reynes J, Rouzier R, Kanouni T, Baillat V, Baroudy B, Keung A, Hogan C, Markowitz M, Laughlin M (2002) Safety and antiviral effects of a CCR5 receptor antagonist in HIV-1-infected subjects. Presented at the 9th Conference on Retroviruses and Opportunistic Infections, Seattle. Abstr 1
84. Rizzardi GP, Morawetz RA, Vicenzi E, Ghezzi S, Poli G, Lazzarin A, Pantaleo G (1998) CCR2 polymorphism and HIV disease. Swiss HIV Cohort. Nat Med 4:252–253
85. Ross TM, Cullen BR (1998) The ability of HIV type 1 to use CCR-3 as a coreceptor is controlled by envelope V1/V2 sequences acting in conjunction with a CCR-5 tropic V3 loop. Proc Natl Acad Sci U S A 95:7682–7686
86. Rucker J, Edinger AL, Sharron M, Samson M, Lee B, Berson JF, Yi Y, Margulies B, Collman RG, Doranz BJ, Parmentier M, Doms RW (1997) Utilization of chemokine receptors, orphan receptors, and herpesvirus-encoded receptors by diverse human and simian immunodeficiency viruses. J Virol 71:8999–9007
87. [Reference deleted in proof]
88. Samson M, Libert F, Doranz BJ, Rucker J, Liesnard C, Farber CM, Saragosti S, Lapoumeroulie C, Cognaux J, Forceille C, Muyldermans G, Verhofstede C, Burtonboy G, Georges M, Imai T, Rana S, Yi Y, Smyth RJ, Collman RG, Doms RW, Vassart G, Parmentier M (1996) Resistance to HIV-1 infection in Caucasian individuals bearing mutant alleles of the CCR-5 chemokine receptor gene. Nature 382:722–725
89. Schols D, Este JA, Cabrera C, De Clercq E (1998) T-cell-line-tropic human immunodeficiency virus type 1 that is made resistant to stromal cell-derived factor 1alpha contains mutations in the envelope gp120 but does not show a switch in coreceptor use. J Virol 72:4032–4037
90. Schols D, Struyf S, Van Damme J, Este JA, Henson G, De Clercq E (1997) Inhibition of T-tropic HIV strains by selective antagonization of the chemokine receptor CXCR4. J Exp Med 186:1383–1388

91. Schuitemaker H, Koot M, Kootstra NA, Dercksen MW, de Goede RE, van Steenwijk RP, Lange JM, Schattenkerk JK, Miedema F, Tersmette M (1992) Biological phenotype of human immunodeficiency virus type 1 clones at different stages of infection: progression of disease is associated with a shift from monocytotropic to T-cell-tropic virus population. J Virol 66:1354–1360
92. Schurmann D, Rouzier R, Nougarede R, Reynes J, Fatkenheuer G, Raffi F, Michelet C, Tarral A, Hoffmann C, Kiunke J, Sprenger H, vanLier J, Sansone A, Jackson M, Laughlin M (2004) Antiviral activity of a CCR5 receptor antagonist. Presented at the 11th Conference on Retroviruses and Opportunistic Infections, San Francisco. Abstract 140LB
93. Sharron M, Pohlmann S, Price K, Lolis E, Tsang M, Kirchhoff F, Doms RW, Lee B (2000) Expression and coreceptor activity of STRL33/Bonzo on primary peripheral blood lymphocytes. Blood 96:41–49
94. Shioda T, Levy JA, Cheng-Mayer C (1992) Small amino acid changes in the V3 hypervariable region of gp120 can affect the T-cell-line and macrophage tropism of human immunodeficiency virus type 1. Proc Natl Acad Sci U S A 89:9434–9438
95. Simmons G, Reeves JD, Hibbitts S, Stine JT, Gray PW, Proudfoot AE, Clapham PR (2000) Co-receptor use by HIV and inhibition of HIV infection by chemokine receptor ligands. Immunol Rev 177:112–126
96. Simmons G, Wilkinson D, Reeves JD, Dittmar MT, Beddows S, Weber J, Carnegie G, Desselberger U, Gray PW, Weiss RA, Clapham PR (1996) Primary, syncytium-inducing human immunodeficiency virus type 1 isolates are dual-tropic and most can use either Lestr or CCR5 as coreceptors for virus entry. J Virol 70:8355–8360
97. Smith MW, Dean M, Carrington M, Winkler C, Huttley GA, Lomb DA, Goedert JJ, O'Brien TR, Jacobson LP, Kaslow R, Buchbinder S, Vittinghoff E, Vlahov D, Hoots K, Hilgartner MW, O'Brien SJ (1997) Contrasting genetic influence of CCR2 and CCR5 variants on HIV-1 infection and disease progression. Hemophilia Growth and Development Study (HGDS), Multicenter AIDS Cohort Study (MACS), Multicenter Hemophilia Cohort Study (MHCS), San Francisco City Cohort (SFCC), ALIVE Study. Science 277:959–965
98. Smyth RJ, Yi Y, Singh A, Collman RG (1998) Determinants of entry cofactor utilization and tropism in a dualtropic human immunodeficiency virus type 1 primary isolate. J Virol 72:4478–4484
99. Speck RF, Wehrly K, Platt EJ, Atchison RE, Charo IF, Kabat D, Chesebro B, Goldsmith MA (1997) Selective employment of chemokine receptors as human immunodeficiency virus type 1 coreceptors determined by individual amino acids within the envelope V3 loop. J Virol 71:7136–7139
100. Strizki JM, Xu S, Wagner NE, Wojcik L, Liu J, Hou Y, Endres M, Palani A, Shapiro S, Clader JW, Greenlee WJ, Tagat JR, McCombie S, Cox K, Fawzi AB, Chou CC, Pugliese-Sivo C, Davies L, Moreno ME, Ho DD, Trkola A, Stoddart CA, Moore JP, Reyes GR, Baroudy BM (2001) SCH-C (SCH 351125), an orally bioavailable, small molecule antagonist of the chemokine receptor CCR5, is a potent inhibitor of HIV-1 infection in vitro and in vivo. Proc Natl Acad Sci U S A 98:12718–12723
101. Takeuchi Y, Akutsu M, Murayama K, Shimizu N, Hoshino H (1991) Host range mutant of human immunodeficiency virus type 1: modification of cell tropism by a single point mutation at the neutralization epitope in the env gene. J Virol 65:1710–1718

102. Tersmette M, de Goede RE, Al BJ, Winkel IN, Gruters RA, Cuypers HT, Huisman HG, Miedema F (1988) Differential syncytium-inducing capacity of human immunodeficiency virus isolates: frequent detection of syncytium-inducing isolates in patients with acquired immunodeficiency syndrome (AIDS) and AIDS-related complex. J Virol 62:2026–2032
103. Theodorou I, Meyer L, Magierowska M, Katlama C, Rouzioux C (1997) HIV-1 infection in an individual homozygous for CCR5 delta 32. Seroco Study Group. Lancet 349:1219–1220
104. Tremblay CL, Giguel F, Hicks JL, Chou TC, Lizawa Y, Sugihara Y, Hirsch MS (2003) TAK-220, a novel small molecule inhibitor of CCR5 has favourable anti-HIV the interactions with other antiretrovirals in vitro. Program and abstracts of the 10th Conference on Retroviruses and Opportunistic Infections, 10–14 February 2003, Boston. Abstr 562
105. Trkola A, Dragic T, Arthos J, Binley JM, Olson WC, Allaway GP, Cheng Mayer C, Robinson J, Maddon PJ, Moore JP (1996) CD4-dependent, antibody-sensitive interactions between HIV-1 and its co-receptor CCR-5. Nature 384:184–187
106. Trkola A, Kuhmann SE, Strizki JM, Maxwell E, Ketas T, Morgan T, Pugach P, Xu S, Wojcik L, Tagat J, Palani A, Shapiro S, Clader JW, McCombie S, Reyes GR, Baroudy BM, Moore JP (2002) HIV-1 escape from a small molecule, CCR5-specific entry inhibitor does not involve CXCR4 use. Proc Natl Acad Sci U S A 99:395–400
107. van Rij RP, Broersen S, Goudsmit J, Coutinho RA, Schuitemaker H (1998) The role of a stromal cell-derived factor-1 chemokine gene variant in the clinical course of HIV-1 infection. Aids 12:F85–90
108. Veazey RS, Klasse PJ, Ketas TJ, Reeves JD, Piatak M Jr, Kunstman K, Kuhmann SE, Marx PA, Lifson JD, Dufour J, Mefford M, Pandrea I, Wolinsky SM, Doms RW, DeMartino JA, Siciliano SJ, Lyons K, Springer MS, Moore JP (2003) Use of a small molecule CCR5 inhibitor in macaques to treat simian immunodeficiency virus infection or prevent simian-human immunodeficiency virus infection. J Exp Med 198:1551–1562
109. Westby M, Smith-Burchnell C, Hamilton D, Mori J, Macartney M, Robas N, Irvine B, Fidock M, Perruccio F, Mills J, Burt K, Barber C, Stephenson P, Dorr P, Perros M (2005) Structurally-related HIV co-receptor antagonists bind to similar regions of CCR5 but have differential activities against UK-427,857-resistant primary isolates. Program and abstracts of the 12th Conference on Retroviruses and Opportunistic Infections, 22–25 February 2005, Boston. Abstr 96
110. Willey SJ, Reeves JD, Hudson R, Miyake K, Dejucq N, Schols D, De Clercq E, Bell J, McKnight A, Clapham PR (2003) Identification of a subset of human immunodeficiency virus type 1 (HIV-1), HIV-2, and simian immunodeficiency virus strains able to exploit an alternative coreceptor on untransformed human brain and lymphoid cells. J Virol 77:6138–6152
111. Winkler C, Modi W, Smith MW, Nelson GW, Wu X, Carrington M, Dean M, Honjo T, Tashiro K, Yabe D, Buchbinder S, Vittinghoff F, Goedert JJ, O'Brien TR, Jacobson LP, Detels R, Donfield S, Willoughby A, Gomperts E, Vlahov D, Phair J, O'Brien SJ (1998) Genetic restriction of AIDS pathogenesis by an SDF-1 chemokine gene variant. ALIVE Study, Hemophilia Growth and Development Study (HGDS), Multicenter AIDS Cohort Study (MACS), Multicenter Hemophilia Cohort Study (MHCS), San Francisco City Cohort (SFCC). Science 279:389–393

112. Wu L, Gerard NP, Wyatt R, Choe H, Parolin C, Ruffing N, Borsetti A, Cardoso AA, Desjardin E, Newman W, Gerard C, Sodroski J (1996) CD4-induced interaction of primary HIV-1 gp120 glycoproteins with the chemokine receptor CCR-5. Nature 384:179–183
113. Zhang Y, Lou B, Lal RB, Gettie A, Marx PA, Moore JP (2000) Use of inhibitors to evaluate coreceptor usage by simian and simian/human immunodeficiency viruses and human immunodeficiency virus type 2 in primary cells. J Virol 74:6893–6910
114. Zhang YJ, Dragic T, Cao Y, Kostrikis L, Kwon DS, Littman DR, KewalRamani VN, Moore JP (1998) Use of coreceptors other than CCR5 by non-syncytium-inducing adult and pediatric isolates of human immunodeficiency virus type 1 is rare in vitro. J Virol 72:9337–9344
115. Zhang YJ, Zhang L, Ketas T, Korber BT, Moore JP (2001) HIV type 1 molecular clones able to use the Bonzo/STRL-33 coreceptor for virus entry. AIDS Res Hum Retroviruses 17:217–227
116. Zhu T, Mo H, Wang N, Nam DS, Cao Y, Koup RA, Ho DD (1993) Genotypic and phenotypic characterization of HIV-1 patients with primary infection. Science 261:1179–1181
117. Zimmerman PA, Buckler-White A, Alkhatib G, Spalding T, Kubofcik J, Combadiere C, Weissman D, Cohen O, Rubbert A, Lam G, Vaccarezza M, Kennedy PE, Kumaraswami V, Giorgi JV, Detels R, Hunter J, Chopek M, Berger EA, Fauci AS, Nutman TB, Murphy PM (1997) Inherited resistance to HIV-1 conferred by an inactivating mutation in CC chemokine receptor 5: studies in populations with contrasting clinical phenotypes, defined racial background, and quantified risk. Mol Med 3:23–36
118. Zou YR, Kottmann AH, Kuroda M, Taniuchi I, Littman DR (1998) Function of the chemokine receptor CXCR4 in haematopoiesis and in cerebellar development. Nature 393:595–599

A Viral Conspiracy: Hijacking the Chemokine System Through Virally Encoded Pirated Chemokine Receptors

H. F. Vischer[1] · C. Vink[2] · M. J. Smit[1] (✉)

[1]Leiden/Amsterdam Center for Drug Research (LACDR), Division of Medicinal Chemistry, Faculty of Sciences, Vrije Universiteit Amsterdam, De Boelelaan 1083, 1081 HV Amsterdam, The Netherlands
smit@few.vu.nl

[2]Department of Medical Microbiology, Cardiovascular Research Institute Maastricht, University of Maastricht, P.O. Box 5800, 6202 AZ Maastricht, The Netherlands

1	Chemokine System	122
2	Viral Immune Evasion	123
3	Herpesvirus-Encoded GPCRs	123
3.1	β-Herpesvirinae	129
3.1.1	Roseoloviruses	129
3.1.2	Cytomegaloviruses	132
3.2	γ-Herpesvirinea	137
3.2.1	Rhadinoviruses	138
3.2.2	Lymphocryptoviruses	141
4	Poxvirus-Encoded GPCRs	142
4.1	Yatapoxviruses, Suipoxviruses, and Capripoxviruses	143
4.2	Avipoxviruses	144
5	Conclusions	144
References		145

Abstract Several herpesviruses and poxviruses contain genes encoding for G protein-coupled receptor (GPCR) proteins that are expressed on the surface of infected host cells and/or the viral envelope. Most of these membrane-associated proteins display highest homology to the subfamily of chemokine receptors known to play a key role in the immune system. Virally encoded chemokine receptors have been modified through evolutionary selection both in chemokine binding profile and signaling capacity, ultimately resulting in immune evasion and cellular reprogramming in favor of viral survival and replication. Insight in the role of virally encoded GPCRs during the viral lifecycle may reveal their potential as future drug targets.

1
Chemokine System

The chemokines and their cognate receptors play a key role in the immune system during homeostasis and inflammation by coordinating leukocyte migration, activation, degranulation, and differentiation. In addition, the chemokine system is involved in organogenesis, angiogenesis, and directing metastasis and growth of tumor cells (Murphy et al. 2000). The mammalian chemokine system (e.g., human, mouse, and rat) constitutes of approximately 45 chemokine ligands and 20 chemokine receptors (Murphy 2002).

Chemokines are a family of small proteins that adopt a similar tertiary folding, even in cases of low overall sequence identity (varying from 20% to 95%). They are characterized by a flexible amino-terminal domain, followed by a conserved core region consisting of a so-called N-loop, three anti-parallel β-strands, and a carboxyl-terminal α-helix, stabilized by disulfide bonds between four conserved cysteine residues (Mizoue et al. 1999). Four subclasses of chemokines (i.e., CC, CXC, CX3C, and XC) have been recognized on the basis of the number and sequential spacing of the first two conserved cysteine residues that are situated near the amino terminus (Zlotnik and Yoshie 2000). In addition, chemokines can be functionally classified into inducible (inflammatory) and homeostatic (constitutively expressed) chemokines, mediating inflammation-directed or basal (homing) leukocyte trafficking, respectively (Proudfoot 2002).

Recruitment of specific leukocyte populations by chemokines is essentially determined by the spatiotemporal expression of selected chemokine receptors, which belong to the membrane-associated G protein-coupled receptor (GPCR) family. Chemokine receptors are classified (i.e., CCR1–11, CXCR1–6, CX3CR1, and XCR1) according to their ability to bind a specific subclass of chemokines (Murphy 2002). Chemokine receptors are not only expressed on leukocytes but also on endothelial, smooth muscle, epithelial, stromal, and neural cells (Onuffer and Horuk 2002). Interestingly, most inflammatory chemokines display a high level of promiscuity by binding several chemokine receptor subtypes, and vice versa. In contrast, homeostatic chemokines are generally more specific, each interacting with a single chemokine receptor subtype (Proudfoot 2002). Given the prominent role of chemokine receptors in regulating intracellular signaling in response to chemokine ligands, these receptors are the most promising targets for immunomodulatory therapeutic interventions (Onuffer and Horuk 2002; Gao and Metz 2003). Interestingly, such receptors are also employed by several viruses in order to subvert the immune system and/or redirect intracellular signaling for their own benefit (Alcami 2003).

2
Viral Immune Evasion

Viruses are small, infectious, parasitic pathogens that (ab)use the host cell metabolism and "consume" cellular biomolecule resources for their replication. An important strategy which enables viruses to replicate efficiently in a host cell is to interfere with recognition and subsequent elimination of the infected cell by the immune system. To this end, distinct viruses have employed different strategies. For instance, large double-stranded DNA viruses, such as herpesviruses and poxviruses, encode viral mimics of host cytokines and chemokines, as well as their soluble binding proteins and/or membrane-associated receptors, to subvert the immune system (Alcami 2003). The viral genes encoding these proteins have probably been derived from the genomes of the viral host during evolution. Of particular interest are the viral genes that code for membrane-associated GPCRs, as these proteins are localized at the boundary of the extracellular and intracellular milieu, and transmit signals from the outside to the inside of the cell. The amino acid sequences of the virally encoded GPCRs (vGPCRs) are generally highly diverged between and within virus subfamilies. This suggests that these GPCRs have distinct and specialized functions that are optimized for different biological properties of each virus. Nonetheless, the majority of vGPCRs display highest sequence similarity to the subfamily of chemokine receptors (Fig. 1, Tables 1 and 2). Some vGPCRs are indeed responsive to chemokines, whereas for others no endogenous ligands have been identified and remain "orphan". Importantly, in contrast to their cellular homologs, a number of vGPCRs signal ligand-independently (i.e., constitutively). Constitutive GPCR signaling is of major significance as revealed by several pathologies associated with activating GPCR mutations (Seifert and Wenzel-Seifert 2002). This constitutive activity of many vGPCRs, together with the current awareness that chemokines and their receptors play prominent roles in inflammatory pathologies and tumor metastases (Proudfoot 2002), suggests that vGPCRs may be key players in virus-associated diseases.

3
Herpesvirus-Encoded GPCRs

Herpesviruses have been isolated from a wide variety of vertebrates and are generally characterized by their strict specificity for a single host species (Davison 2002). Herpesviruses have been classified into three subfamilies, the α-, β-, and γ-herpesvirinae, on the basis of their biological properties,

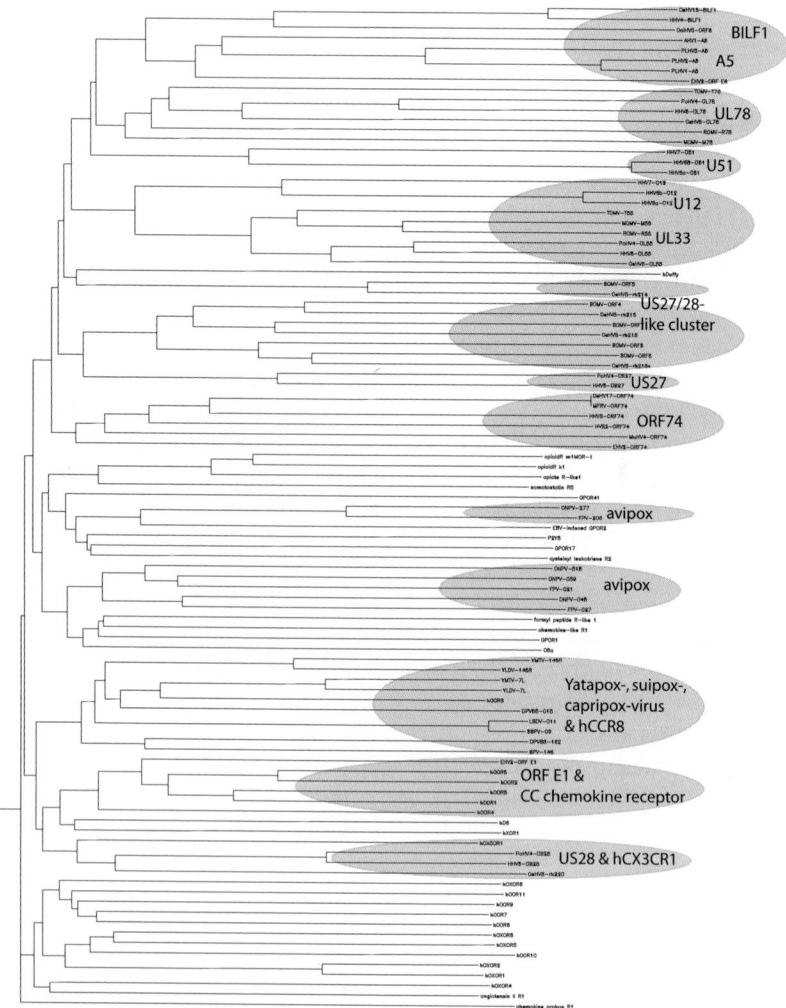

Fig. 1 Phylogenetic relationship between host chemokine receptors and virally encoded GPCRs. Deduced amino acid (reference) sequences of mouse, rat, and human chemokine receptors and vGPCRs were retrieved from the GenBank database at NCBI and analyzed using the ClustalW method (Gonnet series). Chemokine receptor orthologs of mouse, rat, and human all cluster in a single branch per subtype, and are each presented as a single branch for clarity

Table 1 Herpesvirus-encoded GPCRs

Subfamily	Genus	Species		vGPCR	Cellular homolog[a]	%[b]
α-Herpesvirinae	Simplexvirus	Human herpesvirus 1	HHV-1	–	–	–
		Human herpesvirus 2	HHV-2	–	–	–
	Varicellovirus	Human herpesvirus 3	HHV-3	–	–	–
β-Herpesvirinae	Cytomegalovirus	Cercopithecine herpesvirus 8 (Rhesus cytomegalovirus)	CeHV8	UL33	CCR10	20
				UL78	CXCR1	14
				Rh214	CCR5	22
				Rh215	CXCR1	22
				Rh216	CCR1	21
				Rh218	CXCR3	22
				Rh220	CX3CR1	34
		Simian cytomegalovirus (African green monkey cytomegalovirus)	SCMV	ORF3	CCR4	22
				ORF4	CCR3	25
				ORF5	CCR2	22
				ORF6	CXCR1	21
				ORF7	CXCR6	21
		Pongine herpesvirus 4 (Chimpanzee cytomegalovirus)	PoHV4	UL33	CCR3	20
				UL78	CXCR1	13
				US27	CXCR3	23
				US28	CX3CR1	38
		Human herpesvirus 5 (Human cytomegalovirus)	HHV-5	UL33	CCR10	21
				UL78	Somatostatin R3	12
				US27	CXCR3	23
				US28	CX3CR1	36

Table 1 (continued)

Subfamily	Genus	Species		vGPCR	Cellular homolog[a]	%[b]
		Murid herpesvirus 1 (Mouse cytomegalovirus)	MCMV	M33	CCR10	21
				M78	Opiate R-like 1	13
		Murid herpesvirus 2 (Rat cytomegalovirus)	RCMV	R33	CCR10	23
				R78	CCR10	15
		Tupaiid herpesvirus 1 (Tupaia herpesvirus)	TCMV	T33	CCR10	23
				T78	Formyl peptide R-like	12
	Roseolovirus	Human herpesvirus 6a	HHV-6a	U12	CCR10	19
				U51	Cysteinyl leukotriene R2	16
		Human herpesvirus 6b	HHV-6b	U12	CCR10	19
				U51	Cysteinyl leukotriene R2	16
		Human herpesvirus 7	HHV-7	U12	CX3CR1	20
				U51	CCR2	16
γ-Herpesvirinae	Lymphocryptovirus	Callitrichine herpesvirus 3	CalHV3	ORF6	CXCR5	13
			CeHV15	BILF1	CXCR4	14
		Human herpesvirus 4 (Epstein-Barr virus)	HHV-4	BILF1	CXCR4	15
	Rhadinovirus	Alcelaphine herpesvirus 1	AHV1	A5	CCR3	15
		Porcine lymphotropic herpesvirus 1	PLHV1	A5	CXCR2	14
		Porcine lymphotropic herpesvirus 2	PLHV2	A5	CXCR2	15
		Porcine lymphotropic herpesvirus 3	PLHV3	A5	CCR10	13
		Bovine herpesvirus 4	BHV4	–	–	–
		Cercopithecine herpesvirus 17	CeHV17	ORF74	CXCR1	24
		Human herpesvirus 8 (KS-associated herpesvirus)	HHV-8	ORF74	CXCR2	26

Table 1 (continued)

Subfamily	Genus	Species		vGPCR	Cellular homolog[a]	%[b]
		Macaca fuscata rhadinovirus	MFRV	ORF74	CXCR1	24
		Murid herpesvirus 4	MuHV4	ORF74	CCR4	20
		Saimiriine herpesvirus 2 (Herpesvirus saimiri)	HVS2	ORF74	CXCR2	24
		Equid herpesvirus 2	EHV2	ORF E1	CCR3	51
				ORF E6	CCR10	16
				ORF74	CXCR5	22
				ORF E1	CCR3	51

[a] Nearest cellular homologs are identified by basic local alignment search tool (BLAST) analysis of each vGPCR on the human protein sequence reference database at NCBI, subsequently followed by ClustalW analysis
[b] Percentage amino acid identity

Table 2 Chordopoxvirus-encoded GPCRs

Genus	Species	vGPCR	Cellular homolog[a]	%[b]
Avipoxvirus	Fowlpox virus	FPV021	GPCR1	32
		FPV027	GPCR1	29
		FPV206	EBV-induced GPCR2	35
	Canarypox virus	CNPV039	GPCR1	34
		CNPV045	GPCR1	70
		CNPV277	EBV-induced GPCR2	36
		CNPV315	Chemokine-like R1	28
Capripoxvirus	Goatpox virus	GTPV	-	-
	Sheeppox virus	SSPV09	CCR8	40
	Lumpy skin disease virus	LSDV011	CCR8	39
Molluscipoxvirus	Molluscum contagiosum virus	MOCV	-	-
Orthopoxvirus	Camelpox virus	CMPV	-	-
	Cowpox virus	CPV	-	-
	Ectromelia virus	ECT	-	-
	Monkeypox virus	MPV	-	-
	Vaccinia virus	VV	-	-
	Variola virus	VAR	-	-
Parapoxvirus	Bovine papular stomatitis virus	BPSV	-	-
	Orf virus	ORFV	-	-
Suipoxvirus	Swinepox virus	SPV146	CCR8	34
Yatapoxvirus	Yaba monkey tumor virus	7L, 145R	CCR8, CCR8	51, 39
	Yaba-like disease virus	7L, 145R	CCR8, CCR8	53, 44
Unclassified	Mule deer pox	gp013, gp162	CCR8, CCR4	42, 32

[a] Nearest cellular homologs are identified by basic local alignment search tool (BLAST) analysis of each vGPCR on the human protein sequence reference database at NCBI, subsequently followed by ClustalW analysis
[b] Percentage amino acid identity

genome organization, and deduced amino acid sequence similarity between conserved gene orthologs (McGeoch et al. 2000). About 43 genes are shared between most members of the three herpesvirus subfamilies (Davison et al. 2002). These so-called core genes encode proteins that contribute to universal processes such as viral DNA replication and packaging into the viral capsid. During the course of coevolution with their host, individual herpesvirus subtypes acquired unique genes through pirating or gene duplication. Among these so-called accessory genes are genes that allow the virus to subvert the host immune response.

3.1
β-Herpesvirinae

The β-Herpesvirinae subfamily comprises two genera, namely *Roseolovirus* and *Cytomegalovirus* (CMV). Hitherto, four members of the *Roseolovirus* genus have been isolated, three of which are found in man. In contrast, host-specific cytomegaloviruses have been isolated from a wide variety of mammals from the orders Rodentia (e.g., mouse and rat), Scandentia (e.g., tree shrew), and Primates (e.g., rhesus macaque, African green monkey, chimpanzee, and human). CMV genomes are the largest of all herpesviruses (195–241 kb), whereas genomes of roseoloviruses are somewhat smaller (153–162 kb). The genomes of roseoloviruses and CMVs, share extensive characteristics, including position and orientation of large blocks of genes (Neipel et al. 1991; Gompels et al. 1995; Nicholas 1996; Weir 1998).

3.1.1
Roseoloviruses

Three distinct species of *Roseolovirus* have been isolated from peripheral blood of humans. Human herpesvirus (HHV)-6A was first isolated from peripheral blood mononuclear cells derived from adults with acquired immunodeficiency syndrom (AIDS) and displaying lymphoproliferative disorders (Salahuddin et al. 1986). In addition, a second highly related variant of HHV-6, sharing an overall nucleotide sequence identity of 90% (Dominguez et al. 1999), but displaying distinct biological properties, was formally recognized and named HHV-6B. The third human roseolovirus, HHV-7, is highly related to the HHV-6 variants with respect to genome organization as well as sequence, with HHV-6 and HHV-7 genes sharing deduced amino acid identities between 22% and 75% (Nicholas 1996; Dominguez et al. 1999).

Primary infection with HHV-6B occurs between 6 and 12 months of age, whereas infection with HHV-7 occurs at a later time, though often within the first 4 years of childhood (De Bolle et al. 2005). The time of HHV-6A infection is still unknown, but is thought to occur following infection with HHV-6B. As a consequence, roseoloviruses are ubiquitously spread in the general adult population, usually reaching a seroprevalence of greater than 95%. Primary infection with HHV-6b or HHV-7 results in an acute febrile illness that is in some cases followed by the appearance of a mild skin rash on the face and trunk (i.e., exanthem subitum or roseola infantum; Yamanishi et al. 1988; Tanaka et al. 1994). Interestingly, infection with HHV-6A is usually asymptomatic (Dewhurst et al. 1993; Stodberg et al. 2002; Freitas et al. 2003). Clinical complications of (primary) HHV-6 and -7 infections include febrile seizure, but also meningoencephalitis, encephalopathy, and multiple sclerosis (for a review see De Bolle et al. 2005). Importantly, primary HHV-7 infection can reactivate HHV-6 (Frenkel and Wyatt 1992; Katsafanas et al. 1996; Tanaka-Taya et al. 2000). In contrast, reactivation of HHV-6 in healthy children has been reported to occur usually without clinical consequences (Caserta et al. 2004).

Roseoloviruses are (T-)lymphotropic and replicates most efficiently in vitro $CD4^+$ T lymphocytes (Takahashi et al. 1989), but can also infect various other cell types in vitro (De Bolle et al. 2005). HHV-6B and HHV-7 replicate predominantly in salivary glands, with viral shedding into saliva being the major route of virus transmission (Harnett et al. 1990). After primary infection, roseoloviruses persist latently in the host in monocytes and early bone marrow progenitor cells (De Bolle et al. 2005). In healthy individuals, the pathogenic potential of roseoloviruses is kept under control by the immune system. However, both HHV-6 and HHV-7 can reactivate under immunosuppressive conditions (e.g., in AIDS patients and transplant recipients).

The genome of roseoloviruses contains two GPCR-encoding genes, i.e., *U12* and *U51*. The *U12* and *U51* genes are situated on similar positions and have a similar orientation as the *UL33* and *UL78* genes of CMVs, respectively. The *U12* and *U51* genes of HHV-6 are expressed with similar late and early kinetics (Isegawa et al. 1998; Menotti et al. 1999). Temporal expression profiles of the HHV-7-encoded GPCRs have not been reported yet, but are presumably similar to those observed for the HHV-6- and CMV-encoded receptors.

U12 and U51 display the highest amino acid sequence identity to human chemokine receptors. Although the shared sequence identity between these virally encoded receptors and the cellular receptors is rather limited (<20%), both U12 and U51 are highly responsive to a variety of CC chemokines. HHV-6B U12 displays high binding affinity for CCL5, CCL4, and CCL2, and lower affinity for CCL3 (Fig. 2). Moreover, these CC chemokines induce U12-mediated increases in intracellular Ca^{2+} levels in stably transfected K562 cells, via pertussis toxin-insensitive signaling pathways (Isegawa et al. 1998). Interestingly, the HHV-7-encoded U12 displays a different chemokine binding profile than HHV-6B U12 and induces intracellular Ca^{2+} signaling in stably transfected K562 cells in response to CCL17, CCL19, CCL21, and CCL22 (Fig. 2), but not CCL1, CCL2, and CCL5 (Nakano et al. 2003; Tadagaki et al. 2005). In addition, expression of HHV-7 U12 in Jurkat cells induces chemotaxis of these cells towards CCL19 and CCL21 (Tadagaki et al. 2005). Interestingly, CCL17 and CCL22 are unable to attract U12-expressing Jurkat cells. Hence, besides CCR7 and its cognate ligands, U12 expression on the surface of HHV-

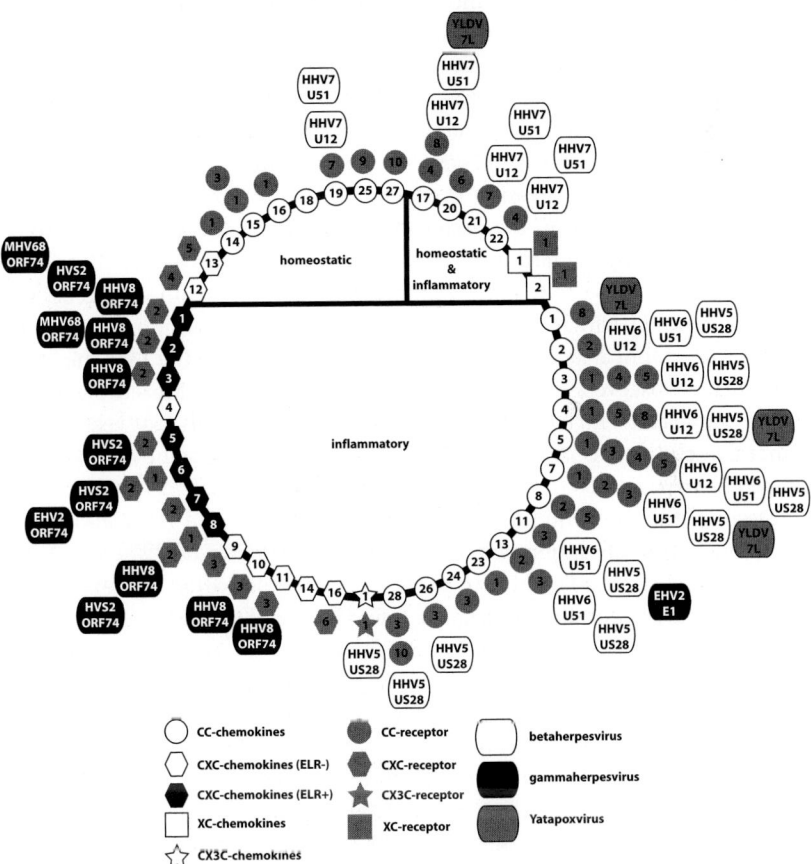

Fig. 2 Chemokine binding of vGPCRs. Homeostatic as well as inflammatory chemokines bind a specific subset of herpesvirus-encoded GPCRs. Chemokines are depicted on the *inner circle*. Their cognate chemokine receptors are displayed next to them, followed by vGPCRs from the β-herpesvirus, γ-herpesvirus, and yatapoxvirus families that were shown to bind the respective chemokines

7-infected T lymphocytes may also support homing of these cells into lymph nodes, which may contribute to viral dissemination.

Despite its low sequence similarity with chemokine receptors, the HHV-6-encoded U51 displays an overlapping chemokine binding profile with HHV-6 U12. This protein binds CCL5 and CCL2 with high affinity, but is unable to bind CCL3. In addition, HHV-6 U51 efficiently binds CCL7, CCL11, CCL13, and HHV-8-encoded viral macrophage inflammatory protein (vMIP)-II (Milne et al. 2000). Interestingly, when transfected into adherent cells (HEK293 or 143tk cells), HHV-6 U51 accumulates predominantly intracellularly in the endoplasmic reticulum and cannot be detected on the cell surface. In contrast, U51 is readily detectable on the cell surface of transfected T lymphocytic cell lines as well as on HHV-6-infected cord blood mononuclear cells in vitro (Menotti et al. 1999). Hence, expression of U51 at the cell surface appears to be cell type-specific, and requires trafficking functions that are apparently present in activated T cells and monocytes, but not in adherent cell types. Interestingly, stable expression of HHV-6 U51 in epithelial cells results in morphological alterations consisting of increased spreading and flattening of the cells and downregulation of CCL5 expression and secretion (Milne et al. 2000). The latter may contribute to immune evasion of the infected cells. The mechanism(s) by which U51 modulates epithelial cell functioning remains to be elucidated, but may include constitutive and/or autocrine U51-mediated signaling as observed for other vGPCRs (Milne et al. 2000). Moreover, in view of the impaired trafficking of U51 to the cell membrane as observed in some adherent cell lines, U51 cell membrane expression needs to be confirmed in epithelial cells.

Despite the low amino acid sequence identity between HHV-7 U51 and U12, these proteins induce intracellular Ca^{2+} elevation in response to the same chemokines (Tadagaki et al. 2005). In contrast, however, U51-expressing Jurkat cells were not able to migrate towards any of the tested chemokines (Tadagaki et al. 2005).

3.1.2
Cytomegaloviruses

Human CMV (HCMV) or HHV-5 is a widely spread virus, with a seroprevalence ranging from 50% to 80%, and it is able to persist lifelong in a latent form. Primary infection of immunocompetent hosts is usually asymptomatic. In contrast, primary infection or reactivation of the virus in immunocompromised hosts, such as the developing fetus, transplant recipients, or AIDS patients, can have severe implications and be fatal (Zhou et al. 1996). Common complications after HCMV infection include damage of liver, brain, retina, and lung (interstitial pneumonitis; Landolfo et al. 2003). Coinfection of HCMV with *human immunodeficiency virus* (HIV) has been shown to accelerate progression to AIDS and dementia in HIV patients (Webster 1991; Kovacs et al. 1999). Increasing evidence suggests that HCMV may also contribute to the development of vascular diseases, e.g., atherosclerosis, restenosis, and vascular allograft rejection (Zhou et al. 1995; Burnett 2001).

CMV primarily infects monocytes, smooth muscle cells, and endothelial and epithelial cells of the upper gastrointestinal, respiratory, or urogenital tracts (Landolfo et al. 2003), and disseminates throughout the body by latently infected monocytes in the blood (Streblow and Nelson 2003). Allogenic stimulation of these monocytes induces differentiation into macrophages, which in latently infected cells is accompanied by reactivation of HCMV leading to the release of infectious virions (Streblow and Nelson 2003). CMV, like other β- and γ-herpesvirus subfamilies, appears to have "pirated" genes encoding key regulatory cellular proteins, showing highest homology to chemokine receptors (Murphy 2001; Sodhi et al. 2004b). HCMV encodes four GPCRs referred to as US27, US28, UL33, and UL78 (Chee et al. 1990). Two GPCR-encoding genes, i.e., *UL33* and *UL78*, are conserved with respect to position and orientation in the genomes of all sequenced β-herpesviruses. Possibly, these genes have been captured from an ancient host species by an ancestral β-herpesvirus. Interestingly, except for the intronless *UL33* genes of rhesus macaque CMV (RhCMV or *cercopithecine herpesvirus 8*) and rat CMV (RCMV), all *UL33* genes consist of two exons interrupted by a single intron. CMV-encoded UL33 orthologs are fairly well conserved and display deduced amino acid sequence identities varying from 35% to 68% (Fig. 1). In contrast, amino acid sequences have diverged considerably between the UL78 orthologs of individual CMV species (12%–54% sequence identity), suggesting a reduced selective pressure on this protein during the course of evolution.

Intriguingly, CMVs infecting host species of the primates (i.e., human, chimpanzee, African green monkey, and rhesus macaque) have pirated an additional GPCR-encoding gene cluster compared with CMVs that infect species from the Glires (i.e., mouse and rat) or Scandentia (i.e., tree shrew) orders. This gene cluster is located in the unique short (US) region of the CMV genome, which is not present in nonprimate CMV genomes, and consists of two adjacent genes in HCMV and chimpanzee CMV (CCMV) (*US27* and *US28*), and five juxtaposed genes in RhCMV and simian CMV (SCMV) (Table 1). Interestingly, the divergence in sequence and number of genes in this gene cluster parallels the coevolution of primate CMVs with two different host species families, with HCMV and CCMV infecting members of the Hominidae family (human and chimpanzee, respectively) and RhCMV and SCMV infecting Old World monkeys (rhesus macaque and African green monkey, respectively). In addition, the highest amino acid sequence identities within proteins encoded by this gene cluster as well as common chemokine binding profiles are observed between rh220, cUS28, and hUS28 (34%–71%), suggesting that these genes have emerged through duplication and rapid diversification of an ancestral US28-like gene.

The genes encoding US28 and UL78 are expressed with early kinetics, whereas *US27* and *UL33* genes are transcribed with late kinetics (Mocarski 1996). The late and early expression kinetics of UL33 and UL78, respectively, are similar to those of their corresponding U12 and U51 counterparts in *Roseolovirus*. In addition, CMV-encoded GPCRs are constituents of the virion, with UL33 (Margulies et al. 1996), UL78 (Oliveira and Shenk 2001), US28, rhUS28.5 (Penfold et al. 2003), and presumably US27 being expressed on the viral envelope. Colocalization of US28 (Fraile-Ramos et al. 2001), US27, and UL33 (Fraile-Ramos et al. 2002) with two major HCMV envelope glycoproteins, i.e., glycoprotein B and H, on virus-wrapping membranes of endocytotic vesicles in transfected or HCMV-infected cells, indicates that these GPCRs are incorporated in the viral envelope.

Although expression of CMV-encoded receptors seems not to be essential for infection of permissive cells in vitro, deletion of either R33/M33 (Davis-Poynter et al. 1997; Beisser et al. 1998) or R78/M78 (Oliveira and Shenk 2001; Kaptein et al. 2003) has significant impact on viral dissemination in vivo. A reduced replication in salivary glands and a lower mortality in infected animals is apparent in in vivo studies using recombinant RCMV and mouse CMV (MCMV) strains, lacking the corresponding *UL33* and *UL78* genes (see Vink et al. 2001 for references), underlining the importance of these receptors in the pathogenesis of infection.

The HCMV-encoded receptor US28 is so far the best characterized HCMV-encoded GPCR. It possesses a large spectrum chemokine-binding profile, including binding of a number of inflammatory CC as well as CX3CL chemokines (Gao and Murphy 1994; Kuhn et al. 1995; Kledal et al. 1998; Penfold et al. 2003; Fig. 2). This broad-spectrum binding profile suggests that US28 could act as a chemokine scavenger and thereby aid in subversion of the immune system (Kuhn et al. 1995; Kledal et al. 1998). CC chemokines, which are shown to bind to US28, induce increasing levels of intracellular calcium, activation of mitogen-activated protein kinase (MAPK) and focal adhesion kinase (FAK). Interestingly, infection of smooth muscle cells with CMV leads a US28-dependent migration. Hence, activation of the former signaling pathways by US28 may provide a molecular basis for the involvement of HCMV in the progression of atherosclerosis. These effects appear to be primarily $G\alpha_{12/13}$ mediated and involve activation of tyrosine kinase-linked signaling pathways (Streblow et al. 2003).

Despite the sequence similarity to chemokine receptors and US28, US27 does not seem to interact with chemokines. Therefore, this receptor is still classified as an orphan receptor. Interestingly, US28 is able to alter cellular signaling in a constitutive manner when expressed in COS-7 cells and after HCMV infection (Casarosa et al. 2001; Casarosa et al. 2003a). US28 is considered a versatile signaling device since it is able to activate multiple signaling networks in a constitutively active manner via activation of effectors and transcription factors within infected cells [i.e., InsP production, nuclear factor (NF)-κB, cAMP-response element (CRE), and nuclear factor activated T cell (NFAT)]. US28 shows promiscuous G protein coupling, through primarily G_q, G_s, and G_{12} proteins (Casarosa et al. 2001; Waldhoer et al. 2002; Casarosa et al. 2003a; Minisini et al. 2003). The chemokine receptor homologs, on the other hand, do not display—or display only limited—ligand-independent signaling and activate primarily $G_{i/o}$ proteins (Offermanns 2003). Interestingly, US28-mediated, constitutive signaling potentiates chemokine-induced signaling of the G_i-coupled CCR1 (Bakker et al. 2004). Since HCMV primarily infects leukocytes, smooth muscle, and endothelial cells—in which chemokine receptors play prominent roles—HCMV-encoded receptor expression may alter ligand-induced signaling via these receptors and contribute to the CMV-induced pathology.

US28-mediated signaling (constitutive or ligand-dependent) is accompanied by G protein receptor kinases (GRK)-mediated phosphorylation of the C-terminal tail, which is followed by a rapid constitutive, agonist-independent endocytosis into perinuclear endosomes and recycling of the receptor US28. The observed internalization of US28 is not dependent on the constitutive activity but involves the C-terminal tail, which serves as a docking site for β-arrestins as well as other scaffolding proteins (Brady and Limbird 2002; Heydorn et al. 2004; Lefkowitz and Shenoy 2005). Binding of these proteins appears important for intracellular signaling and/or receptor trafficking. Interestingly, however, US28 internalization via clathrin-coated pits or lipid rafts is independent of β-arrestins but requires AP-2 adaptor complex proteins and dynamin (Fraile-Ramos et al. 2003; Droese et al. 2004).

CC chemokines do not modulate the constitutive signaling of US28 in the InsP, NF-κB, and CRE assays (Casarosa et al. 2001; McLean et al. 2004), while CX3CL1 acts as inverse agonist in these assays (Casarosa et al. 2001). When US28 loses its capacity to constitutively internalize upon deletion of its C-terminal tail, the CC chemokines, as well as CX3CL1, activate these signaling pathways instead (Waldhoer et al. 2003). Thus, differential modulation of constitutive US28 internalization kinetics and the cellular context in which US28 is expressed determine the efficacy of chemokines acting at this receptor.

The broad chemokine binding profile in combination with rapid and constitutive internalization kinetics (Fraile-Ramos et al. 2001) allows US28 to sequester inflammatory chemokines efficiently from the environment of HCMV-infected cells. As a consequence, the recruitment of leukocytes—and therefore the inflammatory response—may be hampered (Fig. 3; Bodaghi et al. 1998; Billstrom et al. 1999; Randolph-Habecker et al. 2002).

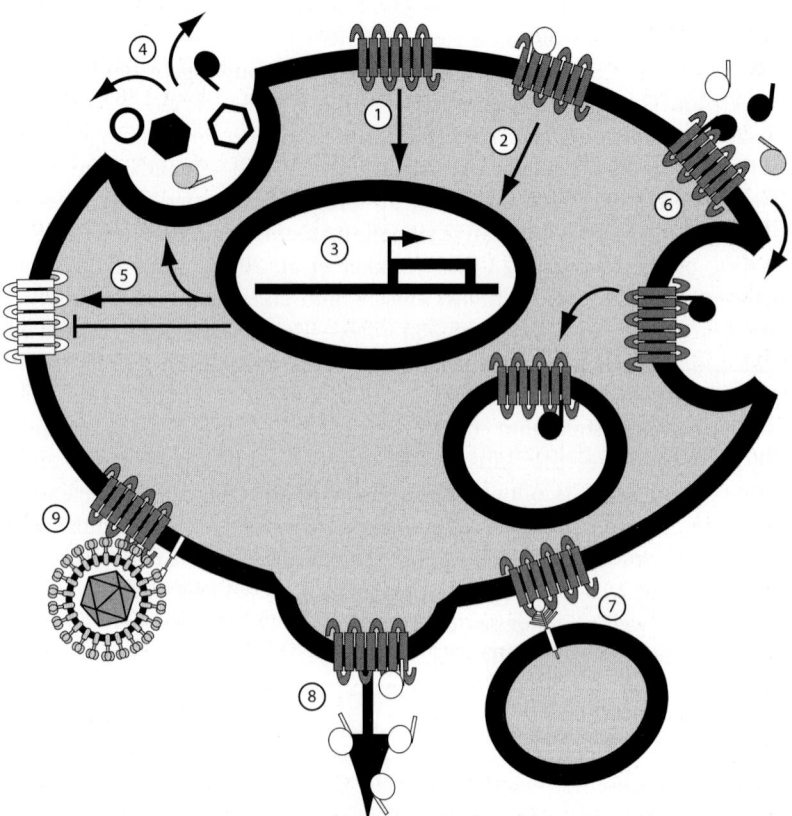

Fig. 3 Suggested roles for vGPCRs. Constitutive (*1*) or ligand-dependent signaling (*2*) of a vGPCR results in up-/downregulation of gene expression (*3*), including autocrine and/or paracrine (angiogenic) factors (*4*) as well as cellular GPCR proteins (*5*). Due to their broad-spectrum chemokine binding profile, vGPCRs may serve as chemokine decoy receptors by internalizing bound chemokine, thereby limiting the immune response (*6*). Binding of vGPCRs (US28) to membrane-associated CX3CL1 facilitates cell–cell adhesion (*7*). vGPCR-mediated chemotaxis in response to chemokine stimulation may increase viral dissemination and other pathogenesis (*8*). In addition, vGPCRs may act as HIV coreceptor (*9*)

The constitutive activity of US28 can be inhibited by a small nonpeptidergic inverse agonist VUF2274 (Casarosa et al. 2003b) derived from a CCR1 antagonist (Hesselgesser et al. 1998). VUF2274 dose-dependently inhibits US28-mediated constitutive activation of phospholipase C in both transfected and HCMV-infected cells, and US28-mediated HIV entry. Importantly, VUF2274 inhibits CCL5 binding in a noncompetitive manner, thus acting as an allosteric modulator. Although a gain in affinity is required, these inverse agonists will serve as valuable tools to further determine the role of (constitutive activity of) US28 in CMV infection.

For UL33, like US28, constitutive signaling has been reported in transfected and infected cells, while no signaling has been detected for UL78 (Casarosa et al. 2003a). Both UL33 and UL78 still remain orphan. In addition, R33 and M33 are able to signal in a constitutively active manner (Gruijthuijsen et al. 2002; Waldhoer et al. 2002). The constitutive signaling of R33 differs from that of UL33 in that R33 is only able to couple to $G_{i/o}$ and G_q, while UL33 shows activation of the G_q, $G_{i/o}$, and G_s classes.

Taken together, CMVs may effectively use their virally encoded receptors to orchestrate multiple signaling networks within infected cells. Importantly, the immediate-early (IE) promoter of HCMV, constituting the genetic switch for progression of viral infection and reactivation, contains four consensus CRE and four NF-κB binding sites. Binding of cognate transcription factors to these sites is required for efficient transactivation of the immediate early promoter (Hunninghake et al. 1989; Keller et al. 2003; DeMeritt et al. 2004; Lee et al. 2004). Moreover, NF-κB is a ubiquitously expressed transcription factor that plays a critical role in the regulation of inducible genes in immune response and inflammatory events associated with e.g., atherosclerosis (Chen et al. 1999). NFAT is an important regulator of immune responses, developmental processes, and angiogenesis (Horsley and Pavlath 2002). It is suggestive to propose that US28 and UL33, through constitutive activation of these transcription factors, induces expression of viral IE proteins and cellular proteins, leading to alteration of the immune response in favor of viral survival and spreading and may contribute by this means to the onset, progression, or enhancement of inflammatory disorders. Further studies in cellular systems more relevant to HCMV infection are required to elucidate the role of these receptors in CMV pathology.

3.2
γ-Herpesvirinea

The γ-Herpesvirinea family is subdivided into the *Lymphocryptovirus* and *Rhadinovirus* genera (Table 1). Although γ-herpesviruses have cell transforming potential, their associated malignancies are mostly seen in the context of immune suppression, such as HIV coinfection or iatrogenic immune suppression, suggesting these viruses are normally "controlled" by the immune system.

3.2.1
Rhadinoviruses

Hitherto, about 48 species of the *Rhadinovirus* genus have been isolated from a wide variety of mammals, of which 8 genomes have been fully sequenced. HHV-8, also known as Kaposi's sarcoma-associated herpesvirus (KSHV), is the only human rhadinovirus identified to date, and was first discovered in Kaposi's sarcoma (KS) skin lesion of an AIDS patient (Chang et al. 1994; Cesarman et al. 1995; Renne et al. 1996). In contrast to the ubiquitous (and infectious) dissemination of most other herpesviruses within their natural host populations, HHV-8 displays a rather low infectivity rate and is unevenly distributed among geographically disparate human populations (Hayward 1999). HHV-8 seroprevalence is low (<5%) in the general population of most European, Asian, and American countries, but can range from 10% to 40% in some Mediterranean countries (Hayward 1999) and 40% to 100% in African countries (Dedicoat and Newton 2003). In addition, HHV-8 seropositivity is highly prevalent among homosexual men (Verbeek et al. 1998). HHV-8 establishes lifelong, latent infections in pre- and post-germinal center B cells and endothelial precursor cells (Dupin et al. 1999), which is characterized by the expression of only a limited number of viral genes (Jenner et al. 2001).

While HHV-8 infection of healthy individuals is usually without severe pathogenic consequences, immune suppression (e.g., in AIDS or transplant recipients) can result in impaired control of HHV-8, leading to multifocal angioproliferative KS lesions (Sturzl et al. 1997) and/or lymphoproliferative diseases (primary effusion lymphomas, multimeric Castleman's disease).

Like other herpesviruses, HHV-8 has captured a cellular gene from its hosts, *ORF74*, which resembles chemokine receptors. The ORF74 receptor shows significant similarity with the human chemokine receptor CXCR2, known to play an important role in angiogenesis, embryonic development, wound healing, and tissue regeneration. Importantly, constitutive expression and signaling of ORF74 induce focus formation in stably transfected NIH3T3 cells, which is accompanied by an increased production and secretion of vascular endothelial growth factor (VEGF), a major angiogenesis activator (Bais et al. 1998). Moreover, these ORF74-expressing cells form highly vascularized tumors that resemble KS when injected into nude mice (Bais et al. 1998). Likewise, transgenic mice expressing HHV-8-encoded ORF74 in hematopoietic or vascular endothelial cells develop angioproliferative KS-like lesions (Yang et al. 2000; Guo et al. 2003; Sodhi et al. 2004c).

ORF74 can constitutively couple to G proteins of the $G_{q/11}$, $G_{i/o}$, and G_{13} classes, thereby modulating a multitude of intracellular signaling pathways, including phospholipases, adenylyl cyclases, kinases, and small G proteins (Arvanitakis et al. 1997; Rosenkilde et al. 1999; Couty et al. 2001; Montaner et al. 2001; Shepard et al. 2001; Smit et al. 2002). Importantly, HHV-8 ORF74-mediated (constitutive) signaling is (partially) increased by angiogenic chemokines [containing a Glu-Leu-Arg (ELR) amino acid motif in the N-terminus]. CXCL8 (ligand for CXCR2) acts as a low-potency partial/neutral agonist (Rosenkilde et al. 1999; Rosenkilde and Schwartz 2000; Couty et al. 2001; Smit et al. 2002; McLean et al. 2004), while the non-ELR, angiostatic chemokines CXCL10 and CXCL12 (ligands of CXCR3 and CXCR4, respectively) and HHV-8-encoded vMIP-II decrease constitutive ORF74 signaling, thus acting as inverse agonists (Fig. 2). Importantly, constitutive signaling by HHV-8 ORF74 as well as chemokine modulation of this constitutive activity are prerequisites for the oncogenic potential of ORF74 in vivo (Holst et al. 2001; Sodhi et al. 2004c). ORF74-mediated modulation of intracellular signaling networks leads to increased transcription of cellular gene and paracrine factors regulating a range of cellular processes including transformation, proliferation, and immortalization (Bais et al. 1998, 2003). HHV-8–ORF74-mediated upregulation and secretion of proangiogenic growth factors and chemokines by lytic cells recruits neighboring cells that can be subsequently infected by released virions (Sodhi et al. 2004a).

Examination of biopsies of KS lesions from AIDS patients revealed high phosphorylated (activated) Akt (PKB) levels, suggesting a critical role for this antiapoptotic serine–threonine kinase in the onset and progression of KS pathology (Sodhi et al. 2004c). Moreover, inhibition of the PI3K/PDK1/Akt pathway prevented proliferation and survival of ORF74-expressing endothelial cells in vitro, and inhibited their tumorigenic potential upon allografting into nude mice (Sodhi et al. 2004c). ORF74 activates Akt by stimulating PI3K through Gβγ-subunits of both pertussis toxin-sensitive and -insensitive G proteins (Montaner et al. 2001), but also via phospholipase C (PLC)-dependent protein kinase C and p44/42 MAPK activation (Smit et al. 2002). In addition, ORF74 activates Akt indirectly in an autocrine manner by upregulating both the expression of VEGF (Bais et al. 1998; Sodhi et al. 2000) and its cognate receptor KDR2 (Bais et al. 2003). Upregulation of growth factors, chemokines, and cytokines in even a few ORF74-expressing cells drives angioproliferative tumor formation by paracrine stimulation of neighboring cells that are latently infected with HHV-8 (Montaner et al. 2003; Jensen et al. 2005). Despite its oncogenic potential, ORF74 is not sufficient for inducing KS in immunocompetent individuals as indicated by one case of KS in every 17,000 HHV-8 infections. ORF74 is primarily expressed during (early) lytic replication, which occurs in about 3% of the spindle-shaped tumor cells within KS lesions (Kirshner et al. 1999; Sun et al. 1999), whereas the majority of cells in KS lesions are latently infected with HHV-8 (Staskus et al. 1997). Moreover, continuous expression of HHV-8–ORF74 appears to be essential for the progression of KS (Jensen et al. 2005). In this respect, it is puzzling how transient expression of HHV-8–ORF74 in lytic cells can cause KS. However, dysregulated expression of ORF74 under certain circumstances—such as HIV-1 coinfection, inflammation, or aborted lytic cycle progression—has been hypothesized to result in non-lytic (continuous) expression of ORF74 in a fraction of KS tumor cells (Sodhi et al. 2004a). In fact, the KS incidence increases about 10,000-fold in HIV-1-infected man, and 100,000-fold in HIV-1-infected homosexual men (Gallo 1998; Reitz et al. 1999), whereas HHV-8-infected transplant recipients have a 500-fold increased risk in developing KS (Cathomas 2003).

In contrast to the ability of HHV-8–ORF74 to constitutively activate a multitude of signaling pathways by coupling to G_q, G_i, and $G_{12/13}$ proteins (Bais et al. 1998; Munshi et al. 1999; Rosenkilde et al. 1999; Sodhi et al. 2000), the ORF74 proteins encoded by nonhuman rhadinoviruses activate a narrower range of G proteins in a ligand-independent manner. Herpesvirus saimiri-encoded ORF74 (i.e., HVS–ORF74 or ECRF3) signals constitutively via G_i and $G_{12/13}$ proteins, but not through coupling to G_q (Rosenkilde et al. 2004). The ORF74 protein encoded by equid herpesvirus 2 (i.e., EHV2–ORF74) only activates G_i-mediated pathways in a constitutive manner (Rosenkilde et al. 2005), whereas ORF74 of murine γ-herpesvirus 68 (i.e., MHV68–ORF74), also known as *murine herpesvirus 4* (MuHV4), is devoid of any constitutive activity (Verzijl et al. 2004). Both constitutive (G_i and $G_{12/13}$) and non-constitutive (G_q) HVS–ORF74-mediated signaling pathways can be stimulated by CXCL1 and CXCL6, whereas CXCL5 and CXCL8 act as neutral antagonists (Rosenkilde and Schwartz 2004). Interestingly, the non-ELR CXC chemokines that act as inverse agonists on the HHV-8–ORF74, do not bind the HVS–ORF74. Likewise, both human and mouse CXCL1 and CXCL2 stimulates MHV68–ORF78-mediated activation PLC, NF-κB, p44/p42 MAPK, and Akt, as well as the inhibition of cAMP formation, whereas non-ELR CXC, CC, and CX3C chemokines were ineffective (Verzijl et al. 2004). In contrast to the broad chemokine binding profile of HHV-8–, EHV2–, and MHV68–ORF74, only a single chemokine (CXCL6) binds to EHV2–ORF74, resulting in a further increase of its constitutive G_i-mediated signaling (Rosenkilde et al. 2005).

Despite the apparent lack of constitutive activity, MHV68–ORF74 expression in NIH3T3 cells induces focus formation by these cells (Wakeling et al. 2001). This transforming potency of MHV68–ORF74 may result from constitutively signaling through yet-unidentified signaling pathways (Verzijl et al. 2004). Alternatively, autocrine secretion of mouse CXCL1 (i.e., KC) by NIH3T3 cells (Bosio et al. 2002) may activate the MHV68–ORF74 that is expressed on the cell surface of these cells. In fact, MHV68–ORF74-mediated signaling in response to mouse CXCL1 enhances in vitro viral replication in permissive NIH3T3 cells (Lee et al. 2003). In contrast, disruption of the MHV68–ORF74 gene did not affect in vitro replication of MHV68 in infected NIH3T12 cells, or in vivo replication in spleen and lungs (Moorman et al. 2003). Interestingly, MHV68–ORF74 appeared to be essential for efficient reactivation of MHV68 from latency (Lee et al. 2003; Moorman et al. 2003). Like other ORF74 genes, *MHV68–ORF74* is an early lytic gene but is also expressed in latently infected cells (Kirshner et al. 1999; Sun et al. 1999; Wakeling et al. 2001).

Interestingly, ORF74-encoding genes are absent in two rhadinoviruses: the *bovine herpesvirus 4* and *alcelaphine herpesvirus 1*. In contrast to other members of the *Rhadinovirus* genus that are sequenced to date, the EHV2 genome contains three additional vGPCR-encoding ORFs adjacent to the conserved ORF74 (Telford et al. 1995). Interestingly, the hitherto uncharacterized ORF E6 displays highest sequence identity to the A5 receptors of *alcelaphine herpesvirus 1* and the lymphotropic porcine herpesviruses 1–3. Moreover, this subfamily of rhadinovirus-encoded GPCRs is homologous to the lymphocryptovirus-encoded BILF1 receptors (see the next section). The other two ORFs are gene duplicates that encode the E1 protein. These ORFs are located in the terminal direct repeat elements on both ends of the genome. E1 displays highest sequence identity to members of the cellular CC chemokine receptor family (30%–51%) and poxvirus-encoded CC chemokine receptors (25%–30%). Despite the relatively high sequence identity with a variety of CC chemokine receptors, only the CCR3-specific chemokine CCL11 was able to induce an E1-mediated increase in intracellular Ca^{2+} levels and chemotaxis (Camarda et al. 1999; Fig. 2).

3.2.2
Lymphocryptoviruses

In contrast to other herpesviruses, lymphocryptoviruses (LCV) have only been isolated from "higher primate" species of the infraorder Simiiformes. Hitherto, about 44 distinct LCVs have been identified (Ehlers et al. 2003). The LCV genomes which have been sequenced include those infecting man [i.e., HHV-4 or Epstein-Barr virus (EBV)], common marmoset [(i.e., *callitrichine herpesvirus 3* (CalHV3)], and rhesus macaques [i.e., *cercopithecine herpesvirus 15* (CeHV15)] have been fully sequenced (Table 1).

LCVs are ubiquitous (>90%) B lymphotropic viruses that establish lifelong, generally asymptomatic, persistent infections in memory B lymphocytes (Wang et al. 2001). However, the potency of LCV to transform B lymphocytes can result in acute infectious mononucleosis, as well as malignant lymphomas, such as Hodgkin's and Burkitt's lymphomas, and post-transplant/AIDS-associated lymphomas (Middeldorp et al. 2003; Thorley-Lawson and Gross 2004). In addition, EBV has been directly associated with nasal natural killer (NK)–T cell lymphoma, nasopharyngeal and gastric carcinoma, oral hairy leukoplakia, and leiomyosarcoma (Middeldorp et al. 2003; Thompson and Kurzrock 2004). Such lymphomas are thought to arise from proliferating, infected B cells that are blocked in the transition from naïve to memory B cells, and/or are not efficiently eliminated by cytotoxic T cells. Hence, individuals with deficiencies in T cell-mediated immunity (e.g., post-transplant immunosuppression and AIDS) are in particular risk of developing EBV-associated lymphoproliferative diseases (Rivailler et al. 2004; Thorley-Lawson and Gross 2004).

The genome of LCVs contains one gene coding for a vGPCR, which is transcribed in various EBV-positive tumor cells (Beisser et al. 2005). LCV-encoded GPCRs show very limited amino acid sequence identity (<15%) to any cellular GPCR (Table 1). Nevertheless, functional analysis revealed that the EBV BILF1 protein is a functional membrane-associated GPCR that constitutively activates NF-κB and CRE signaling pathways—both implicated in cell proliferation—in a G_i-dependent manner (Beisser et al. 2005; Paulsen et al. 2005). In addition, BILF1 constitutively inhibits phosphorylation of the RNA-dependent protein kinase, which is important for antiviral responses (Beisser et al. 2005). Hitherto, BILF1 is still considered an "orphan" receptor, and information on its biological relevance is yet unknown.

4
Poxvirus-Encoded GPCRs

The Poxviridae is a family of large, brick-shaped, double-stranded DNA viruses. A characteristic of these viruses is that they replicate in the cytoplasm of infected cells, independent of the host nuclear machinery. Poxvirus infections are characterized by acute febrile illness accompanied by skin lesions that blister and form pockmarks. Infections are often self-limiting. Some species of poxvirus, however, can cause life-threatening infections in certain hosts (e.g., *variola virus* or smallpox infections in human). Most poxviruses are epitheliotropic and transmitted by direct contact or via the respiratory tract (Diven 2001). Many poxviruses are able to infect a range of host species.

Poxviruses may reside in a reservoir host in which viral infection results in mild, subclinical conditions. However, transfer of the virus to a zoonotic host often causes more severe pathologies (McFadden 2005).

The poxvirus family is divided into the Entomopoxvirinae and Chordopoxvirinae subfamilies, which infect insects or vertebrates, respectively (Table 2). Genome analysis and phylogenetic analysis of multiple deduced amino acid sequences divide the *Chordopox* genera in four (to five) main subgroups (Gubser et al. 2004; see Table 2). Interestingly, the genomes of avipoxviruses, capripoxviruses, suipoxvirus, and yatapoxviruses contain one or more putative GPCR-encoding genes (see Table 2).

4.1
Yatapoxviruses, Suipoxviruses, and Capripoxviruses

The *Yaba-like disease virus* (YLDV) contains two genes, *7L* and *145R*, encoding for membrane-associated proteins that display 53% and 44% amino acid sequence identity with CCR8 (Lee et al. 2001). YLDV-encoded 7L protein, but not 145R, displays a similar chemokine binding profile to CCR8, and binds hCCL1, hCCL7, hCCL4, hCCL17, vMIPI, and vMIPII, but not by mCCL1 (Najarro et al. 2003). In addition, 7L couples to G proteins and induces p44/p42 MAPK phosphorylation in response to CCL1 stimulation. Protein expression analyses of YLDV-infected cells revealed that 7L is expressed as early as 2 h postinfection and its expression increases with time. Blocking late gene expression using a viral DNA replication inhibitor resulted in a 26% decrease in 7L protein expression, suggesting that 7L displays both early and late gene expression kinetics.

The mechanism by which 7L exactly interferes with the CCR8-mediated adaptive and innate immune response has not yet been determined. However, considering the upregulation of CCL1 secretion by dendritic cells, mast cells, and dermal endothelial cells in certain skin inflammations (Gombert et al. 2005), resulting in the recruitment of CCR8-expressing T cells and Langerhans-type dendritic cells, it is tempting to speculate that 7L may sequester CCL1 from the environment of infected cells to impair the immune response. In fact, CCR8 appears to be a vulnerable target for viral hijacking, as several viruses specifically target this receptor by mimicking its ligands (e.g., HHV-8-encoded vMIP-I and vMIP-II, and the molluscum contagiosum virus-encoded vMCC-1) or expressing membrane-associated CCR8 mimics. Alternatively, 7L-mediated signaling in response to CCL1 may also activate anti-apoptotic as well as migratory signaling pathways, as observed for CCR8 (Haque et al. 2001; Louahed et al. 2003; Spinetti et al. 2003; Haque et al. 2004), thereby increasing cell survival and viral dissemination.

Genomes of sui- and capripoxviruses contain a single GPCR gene, of which the deduced amino acid sequences display highest sequence identity to CCR8 (Table 2). However, no pharmacological data are yet available for these receptors.

4.2
Avipoxviruses

The genomes of the fowlpox and canarypox viruses of the Avipoxvirus genus contain 3 and 4 ORFs encoding for vGPCRs. These vGPCRs share about 24% sequence identity with some members of CXC chemokine receptor family, but share more identity with GPCR1 and EBV-induced GPCR2. Nevertheless, this unique cluster of avipoxvirus-encoded GPCRs still awaits functional characterization.

5
Conclusions

Exploitation of the chemokine receptor system through molecular mimicry appears to be an effective means to assist viruses in evading immune surveillance, thus contributing to viral dissemination and virus-induced pathology (Fig. 3). Infection of cells and consequent expression of viral chemokine receptors enables them to respond to a broad spectrum of chemokines, evading the immune response or facilitating viral dissemination to areas with increased chemokine expression (Figs. 2 and 3). The ability of the viral chemokine receptors to signal in a constitutively active manner via promiscuous G protein coupling turns them into versatile signaling devices that modulate cellular signaling networks, thereby reprogramming the cellular machinery to modulate cellular function after infection.

Although many attractive roles have been attributed to this class of receptors, little is known about their (patho)physiological potential. The biological significance of ORF74 and the members of the UL33 and UL78 family in the pathogenesis of HHV-8 and CMV infections has been demonstrated in vivo. Mouse models and studies using recombinant rodent CMVs that carry a disrupted gene or lack the respective gene (Davis-Poynter et al. 1997; Bais et al. 1998; Beisser et al. 1998, 1999; Yang et al. 2000; Oliveira and Shenk 2001; Guo et al. 2003; Kaptein et al. 2003; Sodhi et al. 2004c; Streblow et al. 2005) indicate a role for these viral receptors in pathophysiology. GPCRs constitute a highly drugable class of membrane-associated proteins, accounting for about 50% of protein targets for therapeutic interventions. In addition, the awareness that chemokines and their cognate receptors play a prominent role in numerous pathophysiological processes urges the quest for bioavailable small-molecule antagonists that specifically block viral chemokine receptor functioning (Onuffer and Horuk 2002). Small nonpeptidergic compounds inhibiting US28 constitutive signaling can be considered as tools to investigate the role if US28 in CMV pathology and may serve as promising therapeutics for clinical antiviral intervention. Also for the other viral chemokine receptors, however, specific (pharmacological or RNA interference) inhibitors or antibodies targeting these viral chemokine receptors is essential to elucidate the contribution of viral chemokine receptors to viral pathogenesis and reveal their potential as a future drug target.

Acknowledgements H.F.V. was supported by the Technology Foundation STW, and M.J.S. and C.V. by the Royal Netherlands Academy of Arts and Sciences.

References

Alcami A (2003) Viral mimicry of cytokines, chemokines and their receptors. Nat Rev Immunol 3:36–50

Arvanitakis L, Geras-Raaka E, Varma A, Gershengorn MC, Cesarman E (1997) Human herpesvirus KSHV encodes a constitutively active G-protein-coupled receptor linked to cell proliferation. Nature 385:347–350

Bais C, Santomasso B, Coso O, Arvanitakis L, Raaka EG, Gutkind JS, Asch AS, Cesarman E, Gershengorn MC, Mesri EA, Gerhengorn MC (1998) G protein-coupled receptor of Kaposi's sarcoma-associated herpesvirus is a viral oncogene and angiogenesis activator. Nature 391:86–89

Bais C, Van Geelen A, Eroles P, Mutlu A, Chiozzini C, Dias S, Silverstein RL, Rafii S, Mesri EA (2003) Kaposi's sarcoma associated herpesvirus G protein-coupled receptor immortalizes human endothelial cells by activation of the VEGF receptor-2/KDR. Cancer Cell 3:131–143

Bakker RA, Casarosa P, Timmerman H, Smit MJ, Leurs R (2004) Constitutively active Gq/11-coupled receptors enable signaling by co-expressed Gi/o-coupled receptors. J Biol Chem 279:5152–5161

Beisser PS, Vink C, Van Dam JG, Grauls G, Vanherle SJ, Bruggeman CA (1998) The R33 G protein-coupled receptor gene of rat cytomegalovirus plays an essential role in the pathogenesis of viral infection. J Virol 72:2352–2363

Beisser PS, Grauls G, Bruggeman CA, Vink C (1999) Deletion of the R78 G protein-coupled receptor gene from rat cytomegalovirus results in an attenuated, syncytium-inducing mutant strain. J Virol 73:7218–7230

Beisser PS, Verzijl D, Gruijthuijsen YK, Beuken E, Smit MJ, Leurs R, Bruggeman CA, Vink C (2005) The Epstein-Barr virus BILF1 gene encodes a G protein-coupled receptor that inhibits phosphorylation of RNA-dependent protein kinase. J Virol 79:441–449

Billstrom MA, Lehman LA, Scott Worthen G (1999) Depletion of extracellular RANTES during human cytomegalovirus infection of endothelial cells. Am J Respir Cell Mol Biol 21:163–167

Bodaghi B, Jones TR, Zipeto D, Vita C, Sun L, Laurent L, Arenzana-Seisdedos F, Virelizier JL, Michelson S (1998) Chemokine sequestration by viral chemoreceptors as a novel viral escape strategy: withdrawal of chemokines from the environment of cytomegalovirus-infected cells. J Exp Med 188:855–866

Bosio A, Knorr C, Janssen U, Gebel S, Haussmann HJ, Muller T (2002) Kinetics of gene expression profiling in Swiss 3T3 cells exposed to aqueous extracts of cigarette smoke. Carcinogenesis 23:741–748

Brady AE, Limbird LE (2002) G protein-coupled receptor interacting proteins: emerging roles in localization and signal transduction. Cell Signal 14:297–309

Burnett MS, Gaydos CA, Madico GE, Glad SM, Paigen B, Quinn TC, Epstein SE (2001) Atherosclerosis in apoE knock out mice infected with multiple pathogens. J Infect Dis 183:226–231

Camarda G, Spinetti G, Bernardini G, Mair C, Davis-Poynter N, Capogrossi MC, Napolitano M (1999) The equine herpesvirus 2 E1 open reading frame encodes a functional chemokine receptor. J Virol 73:9843–9848

Casarosa P, Bakker RA, Verzijl D, Navis M, Timmerman H, Leurs R, Smit MJ (2001) Constitutive signaling of the human cytomegalovirus-encoded chemokine receptor US28. J Biol Chem 276:1133–1137

Casarosa P, Gruijthuijsen YK, Michel D, Beisser PS, Holl J, Fitzsimons CP, Verzijl D, Bruggeman CA, Mertens T, Leurs R, Vink C, Smit MJ (2003a) Constitutive signaling of the human cytomegalovirus-encoded receptor UL33 differs from that of its rat cytomegalovirus homolog R33 by promiscuous activation of G proteins of the Gq, Gi, and Gs classes. J Biol Chem 278:50010–50023

Casarosa P, Menge WM, Minisini R, Otto C, van Heteren J, Jongejan A, Timmerman H, Moepps B, Kirchhoff F, Mertens T, Smit MJ, Leurs R (2003b) Identification of the first nonpeptidergic inverse agonist for a constitutively active viral-encoded G protein-coupled receptor. J Biol Chem 278:5172–5178

Caserta MT, McDermott MP, Dewhurst S, Schnabel K, Carnahan JA, Gilbert L, Lathan G, Lofthus GK, Hall CB (2004) Human herpesvirus 6 (HHV6) DNA persistence and reactivation in healthy children. J Pediatr 145:478–484

Cathomas G (2003) Kaposi's sarcoma-associated herpesvirus (KSHV)/human herpesvirus 8 (HHV-8) as a tumour virus. Herpes 10:72–77

Cesarman E, Moore PS, Rao PH, Inghirami G, Knowles DM, Chang Y (1995) In vitro establishment and characterization of two acquired immunodeficiency syndrome-related lymphoma cell lines (BC-1 and BC-2) containing Kaposi's sarcoma-associated herpesvirus-like (KSHV) DNA sequences. Blood 86:2708–2714

Chang Y, Cesarman E, Pessin MS, Lee F, Culpepper J, Knowles DM, Moore PS (1994) Identification of herpesvirus-like DNA sequences in AIDS-associated Kaposi's sarcoma. Science 266:1865–1869

Chee MS, Satchwell SC, Preddie E, Weston KM, Barrell BG (1990) Human cytomegalovirus encodes three G protein-coupled receptor homologues. Nature 344:774–777

Chen F, Castranova V, Shi X, Demers LM (1999) New insights into the role of nuclear factor-kappaB, a ubiquitous transcription factor in the initiation of diseases. Clin Chem 45:7–17

Couty JP, Geras-Raaka E, Weksler BB, Gershengorn MC (2001) Kaposi's sarcoma-associated herpesvirus G protein-coupled receptor signals through multiple pathways in endothelial cells. J Biol Chem 276:33805–33811

Davis-Poynter NJ, Lynch DM, Vally H, Shellam GR, Rawlinson WD, Barrell BG, Farrell HE (1997) Identification and characterization of a G protein-coupled receptor homolog encoded by murine cytomegalovirus. J Virol 71:1521–1529

Davison AJ (2002) Evolution of the herpesviruses. Vet Microbiol 86:69–88

Davison AJ, Dargan DJ, Stow ND (2002) Fundamental and accessory systems in herpesviruses. Antiviral Res 56:1–11

De Bolle L, Naesens L, De Clercq E (2005) Update on human herpesvirus 6 biology, clinical features, and therapy. Clin Microbiol Rev 18:217–245

Dedicoat M, Newton R (2003) Review of the distribution of Kaposi's sarcoma-associated herpesvirus (KSHV) in Africa in relation to the incidence of Kaposi's sarcoma. Br J Cancer 88:1–3

DeMeritt IB, Milford LE, Yurochko AD (2004) Activation of the NF-kappaB pathway in human cytomegalovirus-infected cells is necessary for efficient transactivation of the major immediate-early promoter. J Virol 78:4498–4507

Dewhurst S, McIntyre K, Schnabel K, Hall CB (1993) Human herpesvirus 6 (HHV-6) variant B accounts for the majority of symptomatic primary HHV-6 infections in a population of U.S. infants. J Clin Microbiol 31:416–418

Diven DG (2001) An overview of poxviruses. J Am Acad Dermatol 44:1–16

Dominguez G, Dambaugh TR, Stamey FR, Dewhurst S, Inoue N, Pellett PE (1999) Human herpesvirus 6B genome sequence: coding content and comparison with human herpesvirus 6A. J Virol 73:8040–8052

Droese J, Mokros T, Hermosilla R, Schulein R, Lipp M, Hopken UE, Rehm A (2004) HCMV-encoded chemokine receptor US28 employs multiple routes for internalization. Biochem Biophys Res Commun 322:42–49

Dupin N, Fisher C, Kellam P, Ariad S, Tulliez M, Franck N, van Marck E, Salmon D, Gorin I, Escande JP, Weiss RA, Alitalo K, Boshoff C (1999) Distribution of human herpesvirus-8 latently infected cells in Kaposi's sarcoma, multicentric Castleman's disease, and primary effusion lymphoma. Proc Natl Acad Sci U S A 96:4546–4551

Ehlers B, Ochs A, Leendertz F, Goltz M, Boesch C, Matz-Rensing K (2003) Novel simian homologues of Epstein-Barr virus. J Virol 77:10695–10699

Fraile-Ramos A, Kledal TN, Pelchen-Matthews A, Bowers K, Schwartz TW, Marsh M (2001) The human cytomegalovirus US28 protein is located in endocytic vesicles and undergoes constitutive endocytosis and recycling. Mol Biol Cell 12:1737–1749

Fraile-Ramos A, Pelchen-Matthews A, Kledal TN, Browne H, Schwartz TW, Marsh M (2002) Localization of HCMV UL33 and US27 in endocytic compartments and viral membranes. Traffic 3:218–232

Fraile-Ramos A, Kohout TA, Waldhoer M, Marsh M (2003) Endocytosis of the viral chemokine receptor US28 does not require beta-arrestins but is dependent on the clathrin-mediated pathway. Traffic 4:243–253

Freitas RB, Freitas MR, Linhares AC (2003) Evidence of active herpesvirus 6 (variant-A) infection in patients with lymphadenopathy in Belem, Para, Brazil. Rev Inst Med Trop Sao Paulo 45:283–288

Frenkel N, Wyatt LS (1992) HHV-6 and HHV-7 as exogenous agents in human lymphocytes. Dev Biol Stand 76:259–265

Gallo RC (1998) The enigmas of Kaposi's sarcoma. Science 282:1837–1839

Gao JL, Murphy PM (1994) Human cytomegalovirus open reading frame US28 encodes a functional beta chemokine receptor. J Biol Chem 269:28539–28542

Gao Z, Metz WA (2003) Unraveling the chemistry of chemokine receptor ligands. Chem Rev 103:3733–3752

Gombert M, Dieu-Nosjean MC, Winterberg F, Bunemann E, Kubitza RC, Da Cunha L, Haahtela A, Lehtimaki S, Muller A, Rieker J, Meller S, Pivarcsi A, Koreck A, Fridman WH, Zentgraf HW, Pavenstadt H, Amara A, Caux C, Kemeny L, Alenius H, Lauerma A, Ruzicka T, Zlotnik A, Homey B (2005) CCL1–CCR8 interactions: an axis mediating the recruitment of T cells and Langerhans-type dendritic cells to sites of atopic skin inflammation. J Immunol 174:5082–5091

Gompels UA, Nicholas J, Lawrence G, Jones M, Thomson BJ, Martin ME, Efstathiou S, Craxton M, Macaulay HA (1995) The DNA sequence of human herpesvirus-6: structure, coding content, and genome evolution. Virology 209:29–51

Gruijthuijsen YK, Casarosa P, Kaptein SJ, Broers JL, Leurs R, Bruggeman CA, Smit MJ, Vink C (2002) The rat cytomegalovirus R33-encoded G protein-coupled receptor signals in a constitutive fashion. J Virol 76:1328–1338

Gubser C, Hue S, Kellam P, Smith GL (2004) Poxvirus genomes: a phylogenetic analysis. J Gen Virol 85:105–117

Guo HG, Sadowska M, Reid W, Tschachler E, Hayward G, Reitz M (2003) Kaposi's sarcoma-like tumors in a human herpesvirus 8 ORF74 transgenic mouse. J Virol 77:2631–2639

Haque NS, Fallon JT, Taubman MB, Harpel PC (2001) The chemokine receptor CCR8 mediates human endothelial cell chemotaxis induced by I-309 and Kaposi sarcoma herpesvirus-encoded vMIP-I and by lipoprotein(a)-stimulated endothelial cell conditioned medium. Blood 97:39–45

Haque NS, Fallon JT, Pan JJ, Taubman MB, Harpel PC (2004) Chemokine receptor-8 (CCR8) mediates human vascular smooth muscle cell chemotaxis and metalloproteinase-2 secretion. Blood 103:1296–1304

Harnett GB, Farr TJ, Pietroboni GR, Bucens MR (1990) Frequent shedding of human herpesvirus 6 in saliva. J Med Virol 30:128–130

Hayward GS (1999) KSHV strains: the origins and global spread of the virus. Semin Cancer Biol 9:187–199

Hesselgesser J, Ng HP, Liang M, Zheng W, May K, Bauman JG, Monahan S, Islam I, Wei GP, Ghannam A, Taub DD, Rosser M, Snider RM, Morrissey MM, Perez HD, Horuk R (1998) Identification and characterization of small molecule functional antagonists of the CCR1 chemokine receptor. J Biol Chem 273:15687–15692

Heydorn A, Sondergaard BP, Ersboll B, Holst B, Nielsen FC, Haft CR, Whistler J, Schwartz TW (2004) A library of 7TM receptor C-terminal tails. Interactions with the proposed post-endocytic sorting proteins ERM-binding phosphoprotein 50 (EBP50), N-ethylmaleimide-sensitive factor (NSF), sorting nexin 1 (SNX1), and G protein-coupled receptor-associated sorting protein (GASP). J Biol Chem 279:54291–54303

Holst PJ, Rosenkilde MM, Manfra D, Chen SC, Wiekowski MT, Holst B, Cifire F, Lipp M, Schwartz TW, Lira SA (2001) Tumorigenesis induced by the HHV8-encoded chemokine receptor requires ligand modulation of high constitutive activity. J Clin Invest 108:1789–1796

Horsley V, Pavlath GK (2002) NFAT: ubiquitous regulator of cell differentiation and adaptation. J Cell Biol 156:771–774

Hunninghake GW, Monick MM, Liu B, Stinski MF (1989) The promoter-regulatory region of the major immediate-early gene of human cytomegalovirus responds to T-lymphocyte stimulation and contains functional cyclic AMP-response elements. J Virol 63:3026–3033

Isegawa Y, Ping Z, Nakano K, Sugimoto N, Yamanishi K (1998) Human herpesvirus 6 open reading frame U12 encodes a functional beta-chemokine receptor. J Virol 72:6104–6112

Jenner RG, Alba MM, Boshoff C, Kellam P (2001) Kaposi's sarcoma-associated herpesvirus latent and lytic gene expression as revealed by DNA arrays. J Virol 75:891–902

Jensen KK, Manfra DJ, Grisotto MG, Martin AP, Vassileva G, Kelley K, Schwartz TW, Lira SA (2005) The human herpes virus 8-encoded chemokine receptor is required for angioproliferation in a murine model of Kaposi's sarcoma. J Immunol 174:3686–3694

Kaptein SJ, Beisser PS, Gruijthuijsen YK, Savelkouls KG, van Cleef KW, Beuken E, Grauls GE, Bruggeman CA, Vink C (2003) The rat cytomegalovirus R78 G protein-coupled receptor gene is required for production of infectious virus in the spleen. J Gen Virol 84:2517–2530

Katsafanas GC, Schirmer EC, Wyatt LS, Frenkel N (1996) In vitro activation of human herpesviruses 6 and 7 from latency. Proc Natl Acad Sci U S A 93:9788–9792

Keller MJ, Wheeler DG, Cooper E, Meier JL (2003) Role of the human cytomegalovirus major immediate-early promoter's 19-base-pair-repeat cyclic AMP-response element in acutely infected cells. J Virol 77:6666–6675

Kirshner JR, Staskus K, Haase A, Lagunoff M, Ganem D (1999) Expression of the open reading frame 74 (G-protein-coupled receptor) gene of Kaposi's sarcoma (KS)-associated herpesvirus: implications for KS pathogenesis. J Virol 73:6006–6014

Kledal TN, Rosenkilde MM, Schwartz TW (1998) Selective recognition of the membrane-bound CX3C chemokine, fractalkine, by the human cytomegalovirus-encoded broad-spectrum receptor US28. FEBS Lett 441:209–214

Kovacs A, Schluchter M, Easley K, Demmler G, Shearer W, La Russa P, Pitt J, Cooper E, Goldfarb J, Hodes D, Kattan M, McIntosh K (1999) Cytomegalovirus infection and HIV-1 disease progression in infants born to HIV-1-infected women. Pediatric Pulmonary and Cardiovascular Complications of Vertically Transmitted HIV Infection Study Group. N Engl J Med 341:77–84

Kuhn DE, Beall CJ, Kolattukudy PE (1995) The cytomegalovirus US28 protein binds multiple CC chemokines with high affinity. Biochem Biophys Res Commun 211:325–330

Landolfo S, Gariglio M, Gribaudo G, Lembo D (2003) The human cytomegalovirus. Pharmacol Ther 98:269–297

Lee BJ, Koszinowski UH, Sarawar SR, Adler H (2003) A gammaherpesvirus G protein-coupled receptor homologue is required for increased viral replication in response to chemokines and efficient reactivation from latency. J Immunol 170:243–251

Lee HJ, Essani K, Smith GL (2001) The genome sequence of Yaba-like disease virus, a yatapoxvirus. Virology 281:170–192

Lee Y, Sohn WJ, Kim DS, Kwon HJ (2004) NF-kappaB- and c-Jun-dependent regulation of human cytomegalovirus immediate-early gene enhancer/promoter in response to lipopolysaccharide and bacterial CpG-oligodeoxynucleotides in macrophage cell line RAW 264.7. Eur J Biochem 271:1094–1105

Lefkowitz RJ, Shenoy SK (2005) Transduction of receptor signals by beta-arrestins. Science 308:512–517

Louahed J, Struyf S, Demoulin JB, Parmentier M, Van Snick J, Van Damme J, Renauld JC (2003) CCR8-dependent activation of the RAS/MAPK pathway mediates anti-apoptotic activity of I-309/CCL1 and vMIP-I. Eur J Immunol 33:494–501

Margulies BJ, Browne H, Gibson W (1996) Identification of the human cytomegalovirus G protein-coupled receptor homologue encoded by UL33 in infected cells and enveloped virus particles. Virology 225:111–125

McFadden G (2005) Poxvirus tropism. Nat Rev Microbiol 3:201–213

McGeoch DJ, Dolan A, Ralph AC (2000) Toward a comprehensive phylogeny for mammalian and avian herpesviruses. J Virol 74:10401–10406

McLean KA, Holst PJ, Martini L, Schwartz TW, Rosenkilde MM (2004) Similar activation of signal transduction pathways by the herpesvirus-encoded chemokine receptors US28 and ORF74. Virology 325:241–251

Menotti L, Mirandola P, Locati M, Campadelli-Fiume G (1999) Trafficking to the plasma membrane of the seven-transmembrane protein encoded by human herpesvirus 6 U51 gene involves a cell-specific function present in T lymphocytes. J Virol 73:325–333

Middeldorp JM, Brink AA, van den Brule AJ, Meijer CJ (2003) Pathogenic roles for Epstein-Barr virus (EBV) gene products in EBV-associated proliferative disorders. Crit Rev Oncol Hematol 45:1–36

Milne RS, Mattick C, Nicholson L, Devaraj P, Alcami A, Gompels UA (2000) RANTES binding and down-regulation by a novel human herpesvirus-6 beta chemokine receptor. J Immunol 164:2396–2404

Minisini R, Tulone C, Luske A, Michel D, Mertens T, Gierschik P, Moepps B (2003) Constitutive inositol phosphate formation in cytomegalovirus-infected human fibroblasts is due to expression of the chemokine receptor homologue pUS28. J Virol 77:4489–4501

Mizoue LS, Bazan JF, Johnson EC, Handel TM (1999) Solution structure and dynamics of the CX3C chemokine domain of fractalkine and its interaction with an N-terminal fragment of CX3CR1. Biochemistry 38:1402–1414

Mocarski ES (1996) Cytomegalovirus and their replication. In: Fields BN, Knipe DM, Howley PM (eds) Fields virology. Lippincott-Raven, Philadelphia, pp 2447–2492

Montaner S, Sodhi A, Pece S, Mesri EA, Gutkind JS (2001) The Kaposi's sarcoma-associated herpesvirus G protein-coupled receptor promotes endothelial cell survival through the activation of Akt/protein kinase B. Cancer Res 61:2641–2648

Montaner S, Sodhi A, Molinolo A, Bugge TH, Sawai ET, He Y, Li Y, Ray PE, Gutkind JS (2003) Endothelial infection with KSHV genes in vivo reveals that vGPCR initiates Kaposi's sarcomagenesis and can promote the tumorigenic potential of viral latent genes. Cancer Cell 3:23–36

Moorman NJ, Virgin HWt, Speck SH (2003) Disruption of the gene encoding the gammaHV68 v-GPCR leads to decreased efficiency of reactivation from latency. Virology 307:179–190

Munshi N, Ganju RK, Avraham S, Mesri EA, Groopman JE (1999) Kaposi's sarcoma-associated herpesvirus-encoded G protein-coupled receptor activation of c-jun amino-terminal kinase/stress-activated protein kinase and lyn kinase is mediated by related adhesion focal tyrosine kinase/proline-rich tyrosine kinase 2. J Biol Chem 274:31863–31867

Murphy PM (2001) Viral exploitation and subversion of the immune system through chemokine mimicry. Nat Immunol 2:116–122

Murphy PM (2002) International Union of Pharmacology. XXX. Update on chemokine receptor nomenclature. Pharmacol Rev 54:227–229

Murphy PM, Baggiolini M, Charo IF, Hebert CA, Horuk R, Matsushima K, Miller LH, Oppenheim JJ, Power CA (2000) International union of pharmacology. XXII Nomenclature for chemokine receptors. Pharmacol Rev 52:145–176

Najarro P, Lee HJ, Fox J, Pease J, Smith GL (2003) Yaba-like disease virus protein 7L is a cell-surface receptor for chemokine CCL1. J Gen Virol 84:3325–3336

Nakano K, Tadagaki K, Isegawa Y, Aye MM, Zou P, Yamanishi K (2003) Human herpesvirus 7 open reading frame U12 encodes a functional beta-chemokine receptor. J Virol 77:8108–8115

Neipel F, Ellinger K, Fleckenstein B (1991) The unique region of the human herpesvirus 6 genome is essentially collinear with the UL segment of human cytomegalovirus. J Gen Virol 72:2293–2297

Nicholas J (1996) Determination and analysis of the complete nucleotide sequence of human herpesvirus. J Virol 70:5975–5989

Offermanns S (2003) G-proteins as transducers in transmembrane signalling. Prog Biophys Mol Biol 83:101–130

Oliveira SA, Shenk TE (2001) Murine cytomegalovirus M78 protein, a G protein-coupled receptor homologue, is a constituent of the virion and facilitates accumulation of immediate-early viral mRNA. Proc Natl Acad Sci U S A 98:3237–3242

Onuffer JJ, Horuk R (2002) Chemokines, chemokine receptors and small-molecule antagonists: recent developments. Trends Pharmacol Sci 23:459–467

Paulsen SJ, Rosenkilde MM, Eugen-Olsen J, Kledal TN (2005) Epstein-Barr virus-encoded BILF1 is a constitutively active G protein-coupled receptor. J Virol 79:536–546

Penfold ME, Schmidt TL, Dairaghi DJ, Barry PA, Schall TJ (2003) Characterization of the rhesus cytomegalovirus US28 locus. J Virol 77:10404–10413

Proudfoot AE (2002) Chemokine receptors: multifaceted therapeutic targets. Nat Rev Immunol 2:106–115

Randolph-Habecker JR, Rahill B, Torok-Storb B, Vieira J, Kolattukudy PE, Rovin BH, Sedmak DD (2002) The expression of the cytomegalovirus chemokine receptor homolog US28 sequesters biologically active CC chemokines and alters IL-8 production. Cytokine 19:37–46

Reitz MS Jr, Nerurkar LS, Gallo RC (1999) Perspective on Kaposi's sarcoma: facts, concepts, and conjectures. J Natl Cancer Inst 91:1453–1458

Renne R, Zhong W, Herndier B, McGrath M, Abbey N, Kedes D, Ganem D (1996) Lytic growth of Kaposi's sarcoma-associated herpesvirus (human herpesvirus 8) in culture. Nat Med 2:342–346

Rivailler P, Carville A, Kaur A, Rao P, Quink C, Kutok JL, Westmoreland S, Klumpp S, Simon M, Aster JC, Wang F (2004) Experimental rhesus lymphocryptovirus infection in immunosuppressed macaques: an animal model for Epstein-Barr virus pathogenesis in the immunosuppressed host. Blood 104:1482–1489

Rosenkilde MM, Schwartz TW (2000) Potency of ligands correlates with affinity measured against agonist and inverse agonists but not against neutral ligand in constitutively active chemokine receptor. Mol Pharmacol 57:602–609

Rosenkilde MM, Schwartz TW (2004) The chemokine system—a major regulator of angiogenesis in health and disease. Apmis 112:481–495

Rosenkilde MM, Kledal TN, Brauner-Osborne H, Schwartz TW (1999) Agonists and inverse agonists for the herpesvirus 8-encoded constitutively active seven-transmembrane oncogene product, ORF-74. J Biol Chem 274:956–961

Rosenkilde MM, McLean KA, Holst PJ, Schwartz TW (2004) The CXC chemokine receptor encoded by herpesvirus saimiri, ECRF3, shows ligand-regulated signaling through Gi, Gq, and G12/13 proteins but constitutive signaling only through Gi and G12/13 proteins. J Biol Chem 279:32524–32533

Rosenkilde MM, Kledal TN, Schwartz TW (2005) High constitutive activity of a virus-encoded seven transmembrane receptor in the absence of the conserved DRY motif (Asp-Arg-Tyr) in transmembrane helix 3. Mol Pharmacol 68:11–19

Salahuddin SZ, Ablashi DV, Markham PD, Josephs SF, Sturzenegger S, Kaplan M, Halligan G, Biberfeld P, Wong-Staal F, Kramarsky B, et al (1986) Isolation of a new virus, HBLV, in patients with lymphoproliferative disorders. Science 234:596–601

Seifert R, Wenzel-Seifert K (2002) Constitutive activity of G-protein-coupled receptors: cause of disease and common property of wild-type receptors. Naunyn Schmiedebergs Arch Pharmacol 366:381–416

Shepard LW, Yang M, Xie P, Browning DD, Voyno-Yasenetskaya T, Kozasa T, Ye RD (2001) Constitutive activation of NF-kappa B and secretion of interleukin-8 induced by the G protein-coupled receptor of Kaposi's sarcoma-associated herpesvirus involve G alpha(13) and RhoA. J Biol Chem 276:45979–45987

Smit MJ, Verzijl D, Casarosa P, Navis M, Timmerman H, Leurs R (2002) Kaposi's sarcoma-associated herpesvirus-encoded G protein-coupled receptor ORF74 constitutively activates p44/p42 MAPK and Akt via G(i) and phospholipase C-dependent signaling pathways. J Virol 76:1744–1752

Sodhi A, Montaner S, Patel V, Zohar M, Bais C, Mesri EA, Gutkind JS (2000) The Kaposi's sarcoma-associated herpes virus G protein-coupled receptor up-regulates vascular endothelial growth factor expression and secretion through mitogen-activated protein kinase and p38 pathways acting on hypoxia-inducible factor 1alpha. Cancer Res 60:4873–4880

Sodhi A, Montaner S, Gutkind JS (2004a) Does dysregulated expression of a deregulated viral GPCR trigger Kaposi's sarcomagenesis? Faseb J 18:422–427

Sodhi A, Montaner S, Gutkind JS (2004b) Viral hijacking of G-protein-coupled-receptor signalling networks. Nat Rev Mol Cell Biol 5:998–1012

Sodhi A, Montaner S, Patel V, Gomez-Roman JJ, Li Y, Sausville EA, Sawai ET, Gutkind JS (2004c) Akt plays a central role in sarcomagenesis induced by Kaposi's sarcoma herpesvirus-encoded G protein-coupled receptor. Proc Natl Acad Sci U S A 101:4821–4826

Spinetti G, Bernardini G, Camarda G, Mangoni A, Santoni A, Capogrossi MC, Napolitano M (2003) The chemokine receptor CCR8 mediates rescue from dexamethasone-induced apoptosis via an ERK-dependent pathway. J Leukoc Biol 73:201–207

Staskus KA, Zhong W, Gebhard K, Herndier B, Wang H, Renne R, Beneke J, Pudney J, Anderson DJ, Ganem D, Haase AT (1997) Kaposi's sarcoma-associated herpesvirus gene expression in endothelial (spindle) tumor cells. J Virol 71:715–719

Stodberg T, Deniz Y, Esteitie N, Jacobsson B, Mousavi-Jazi M, Dahl H, Zweygberg Wirgart B, Grillner L, Linde A (2002) A case of diffuse leptomeningeal oligodendrogliomatosis associated with HHV-6 variant A. Neuropediatrics 33:266–270

Streblow DN, Nelson JA (2003) Models of HCMV latency and reactivation. Trends Microbiol 11:293–295

Streblow DN, Vomaske J, Smith P, Melnychuk R, Hall L, Pancheva D, Smit M, Casarosa P, Schlaepfer DD, Nelson JA (2003) Human cytomegalovirus chemokine receptor US28-induced smooth muscle cell migration is mediated by focal adhesion kinase and Src. J Biol Chem 278:50456–50465

Streblow DN, Kreklywich CN, Smith P, Soule JL, Meyer C, Yin M, Beisser P, Vink C, Nelson JA, Orloff SL (2005) Rat cytomegalovirus-accelerated transplant vascular sclerosis is reduced with mutation of the chemokine-receptor R33. Am J Transplant 5:436–442

Sturzl M, Blasig C, Schreier A, Neipel F, Hohenadl C, Cornali E, Ascherl G, Esser S, Brockmeyer NH, Ekman M, Kaaya EE, Tschachler E, Biberfeld P (1997) Expression of HHV-8 latency-associated T0.7 RNA in spindle cells and endothelial cells of AIDS-associated, classical and African Kaposi's sarcoma. Int J Cancer 72:68–71

Sun R, Lin SF, Staskus K, Gradoville L, Grogan E, Haase A, Miller G (1999) Kinetics of Kaposi's sarcoma-associated herpesvirus gene expression. J Virol 73:2232–2242

Tadagaki K, Nakano K, Yamanishi K (2005) Human herpesvirus 7 open reading frames U12 and U51 encode functional beta-chemokine receptors. J Virol 79:7068–7076

Takahashi K, Sonoda S, Higashi K, Kondo T, Takahashi H, Takahashi M, Yamanishi K (1989) Predominant CD4 T-lymphocyte tropism of human herpesvirus 6-related virus. J Virol 63:3161–3163

Tanaka K, Kondo T, Torigoe S, Okada S, Mukai T, Yamanishi K (1994) Human herpesvirus 7: another causal agent for roseola (exanthem subitum). J Pediatr 125:1–5

Tanaka-Taya K, Kondo T, Nakagawa N, Inagi R, Miyoshi H, Sunagawa T, Okada S, Yamanishi K (2000) Reactivation of human herpesvirus 6 by infection of human herpesvirus 7. J Med Virol 60:284–289

Telford EA, Watson MS, Aird HC, Perry J, Davison AJ (1995) The DNA sequence of equine herpesvirus 2. J Mol Biol 249:520–528

Thompson MP, Kurzrock R (2004) Epstein-Barr virus and cancer. Clin Cancer Res 10:803–821

Thorley-Lawson DA, Gross A (2004) Persistence of the Epstein-Barr virus and the origins of associated lymphomas. N Engl J Med 350:1328–1337

Verbeek W, Frankel M, Miles S, Said J, Koeffler HP (1998) Seroprevalence of HHV-8 antibodies in HIV-positive homosexual men without Kaposi's sarcoma and their clinical follow-up. Am J Clin Pathol 109:778-783

Verzijl D, Fitzsimons CP, Van Dijk M, Stewart JP, Timmerman H, Smit MJ, Leurs R (2004) Differential activation of murine herpesvirus 68- and Kaposi's sarcoma-associated herpesvirus-encoded ORF74 G protein-coupled receptors by human and murine chemokines. J Virol 78:3343-3351

Vink C, Smit MJ, Leurs R, Bruggeman CA (2001) The role of cytomegalovirus-encoded homologs of G protein-coupled receptors and chemokines in manipulation of and evasion from the immune system. J Clin Virol 23:43-55

Wakeling MN, Roy DJ, Nash AA, Stewart JP (2001) Characterization of the murine gammaherpesvirus 68 ORF74 product: a novel oncogenic G protein-coupled receptor. J Gen Virol 82:1187-1197

Waldhoer M, Kledal TN, Farrell H, Schwartz TW (2002) Murine cytomegalovirus (CMV) M33 and human CMV US28 receptors exhibit similar constitutive signaling activities. J Virol 76:8161-8168

Waldhoer M, Casarosa P, Rosenkilde MM, Smit MJ, Leurs R, Whistler JL, Schwartz TW (2003) The carboxyl terminus of human cytomegalovirus-encoded 7 transmembrane receptor US28 camouflages agonism by mediating constitutive endocytosis. J Biol Chem 278:19473-19482

Wang F, Rivailler P, Rao P, Cho Y (2001) Simian homologues of Epstein-Barr virus. Philos Trans R Soc Lond B Biol Sci 356:489-497

Webster A (1991) Cytomegalovirus as a possible cofactor in HIV disease progression. J Acquir Immune Defic Syndr 4:S47-S52

Weir JP (1998) Genomic organization and evolution of the human herpesviruses. Virus Genes 16:85-93

Yamanishi K, Okuno T, Shiraki K, Takahashi M, Kondo T, Asano Y, Kurata T (1988) Identification of human herpesvirus-6 as a causal agent for exanthem subitum. Lancet 1:1065-1067

Yang TY, Chen SC, Leach MW, Manfra D, Homey B, Wiekowski M, Sullivan L, Jenh CH, Narula SK, Chensue SW, Lira SA (2000) Transgenic expression of the chemokine receptor encoded by human herpesvirus 8 induces an angioproliferative disease resembling Kaposi's sarcoma. J Exp Med 191:445-454

Zhou YF, Shou M, Guzman R, Guetta E, Finkel T, Epstein SE (1995) Cytomegalovirus infection increases neointimal formation in the rat model of balloon injury. J Am Coll Cardiol 25:242a

Zhou YF, Leon MB, Waclawiw MA, Popma JJ, Yu ZX, Finkel T, Epstein SE (1996) Association between prior cytomegalovirus infection and the risk of restenosis after coronary atherectomy. N Engl J Med 335:624-630

Zlotnik A, Yoshie O (2000) Chemokines: a new classification system and their role in immunity. Immunity 12:121-127

Subject Index

adoptive transfer 11
AK602/GSK-873140 107
alternative coreceptor 100
AMD-070 108
AMD-3100 108
antibody 4
apoptosis 71, 75, 82, 83, 86, 87
astrocytes 4, 70, 75, 76, 78–80, 84–87

BILF1 141, 142
blood–brain barrier 81

caprine arthritis encephalitis virus (CAEV) 69, 70
CCL12 77, 78
CCL2 6, 76–84, 86
Ccl2 73
CCL22 82, 83
CCL3 6, 76–80, 82, 83, 85
Ccl3 73
CCL4 6, 76–79, 82, 85
Ccl4 73
CCL5 6, 76–79, 82, 83, 85
Ccl5 73
CCL7 6, 77–79, 86
CCR1 6, 83, 84, 86
CCR10 84
CCR2 6, 78, 80, 81, 83–85
CCR2-64I polymorphism 102
CCR5 6, 78, 82–86, 100, 101
CCR5 59029 G/A single-nucleotide polymorphism 102
CCR5 Δ32 101, 103
CD4 98
– role as HIV receptor 98

$CD4^+$ T cells 4
$CD8^+$ lymphocytes 81, 82
$CD8^+$ T cells 3
chemokine receptor 6, 83–86
CMPD 167 106
coronaviruses 2
coxsackievirus 9
CXCL10 6, 76, 77, 79, 80, 83, 84
Cxcl10 73
CXCL12 82–84
CXCL9 6, 80
CXCR3 6, 83
CXCR4 82, 84–86, 100

dendritic cells (DCs) 8

ECRF3 *see* HVS-ORF74
EHV2-ORF74 140
enfuvirtide 110
envelope 73, 74, 80, 83, 85
epitope spreading 5
equine infectious anemia virus 70

feline immunodeficiency virus (FIV) 69, 71, 72, 77, 79–81, 84, 86
fractalkine 5
FrCasE 69–71, 79

γδ T cells 5

HHV-8ORF74 *see* ORF74
HIV 69–71, 77, 79–86
HIV Tat 80, 82, 86
HIV tropism 98
– M-tropic 100
– T-tropic 100

human T cell leukemia virus (HTLV) 69, 70
HVS–ORF74   140

IL-1   79
$IL\text{-}1\alpha$ 73
IL-1α   86
IL-1β   80
IL-4   79
IL-6   79
influenza virus   9
interferon (IFN)-γ   4, 79

7L   143
lymphocytes   71, 79, 81, 86
lymphotactin   5

M33   134, 137
M78   134
macrophages   4, 70, 71, 75, 76, 78, 79, 81, 82, 85–87
MHV68–ORF74   140, 141
microglia   4, 70, 71, 73, 75, 76, 78–81, 85, 86
MIP-1α   100, 103, 105, 107
MIP-1β   100, 103, 105, 107
Mol-ts1   70, 79
Moloney-ts1   69
multiple sclerosis (MS)   4

neurons   69, 70, 82–84, 86
neuroprogenitor stem cell   83
- migration   87

oligodendrocytes   70, 73
ORF74   138, 140
- angiogenesis   138, 139
- chemokine-induced signaling   139
- constitutive signaling   139, 140
- CXC-chemokine   139
- expression   140, 141
- Kaposi's sarcoma   138–140
- oncogene   139
- vascular endothelial growth factor (VEGF)   138, 139

paramyxovirus   9
progression to AIDS   100, 102, 103

145R   143
R33   134, 137
R78   134
$RAG1^{-/-}$ mice   4
RANTES   100, 103, 105, 107
- derivatives of RANTES   103
receptor US28   134
resistance to coreceptor inhibitor   108

SCH-C   105
SCH-D   106
SDF-1α   100, 107
SDF-1β   100, 102
secondary lymphoid organs   10
SIV   69–72, 77, 79–82, 84–86

TAK-220   105
TAK-652   105
TAK-779   104
Theiler's virus   5
TR1.3   70, 71
tumor necrosis factor (TNF)   73, 76–82, 85, 86
tumor necrosis factor receptor I (TNFRI)   79, 82
tumor necrosis factor receptor I (TNFRII)   82
type I interferons   7

U12   130–132
U51   130, 132
UK-427857   106
UL33   130, 133, 134, 137
UL78   130, 133, 134, 137
US27   133–135
US28   133–135, 137
- allosteric modulator   137
- CC-chemokine   134, 135
- chemokine binding   134, 136, 137
- chemokine-induced signaling   135

- chemotaxis   134
- constitutive signaling   135, 137
- CX3CL-chemokine   134, 135
- endocytosis   135
- expression   134
- gene   133, 134
- HIV coreceptor   137
- internalization   135, 136
- migration   134
- protein localization   134

V3 loop   101
- primary determinant of viral tropism   101

visna   69, 70

xenotropic/polytropic receptor   86

Current Topics in Microbiology and Immunology

Volumes published since 1989 (and still available)

Vol. 259: **Hauber, Joachim, Vogt, Peter K. (Eds.):** Nuclear Export of Viral RNAs. 2001. 19 figs. IX, 131 pp. ISBN 3-540-41278-6

Vol. 260: **Burton, Didier R. (Ed.):** Antibodies in Viral Infection. 2001. 51 figs. IX, 309 pp. ISBN 3-540-41611-0

Vol. 261: **Trono, Didier (Ed.):** Lentiviral Vectors. 2002. 32 figs. X, 258 pp. ISBN 3-540-42190-4

Vol. 262: **Oldstone, Michael B.A. (Ed.):** Arenaviruses I. 2002. 30 figs. XVIII, 197 pp. ISBN 3-540-42244-7

Vol. 263: **Oldstone, Michael B. A. (Ed.):** Arenaviruses II. 2002. 49 figs. XVIII, 268 pp. ISBN 3-540-42705-8

Vol. 264/I: **Hacker, Jörg; Kaper, James B. (Eds.):** Pathogenicity Islands and the Evolution of Microbes. 2002. 34 figs. XVIII, 232 pp. ISBN 3-540-42681-7

Vol. 264/II: **Hacker, Jörg; Kaper, James B. (Eds.):** Pathogenicity Islands and the Evolution of Microbes. 2002. 24 figs. XVIII, 228 pp. ISBN 3-540-42682-5

Vol. 265: **Dietzschold, Bernhard; Richt, Jürgen A. (Eds.):** Protective and Pathological Immune Responses in the CNS. 2002. 21 figs. X, 278 pp. ISBN 3-540-42668X

Vol. 266: **Cooper, Koproski (Eds.):** The Interface Between Innate and Acquired Immunity, 2002. 15 figs. XIV, 116 pp. ISBN 3-540-42894-X

Vol. 267: **Mackenzie, John S.; Barrett, Alan D. T.; Deubel, Vincent (Eds.):** Japanese Encephalitis and West Nile Viruses. 2002. 66 figs. X, 418 pp. ISBN 3-540-42783X

Vol. 268: **Zwickl, Peter; Baumeister, Wolfgang (Eds.):** The Proteasome-Ubiquitin Protein Degradation Pathway. 2002. 17 figs. X, 213 pp. ISBN 3-540-43096-2

Vol. 269: **Koszinowski, Ulrich H.; Hengel, Hartmut (Eds.):** Viral Proteins Counteracting Host Defenses. 2002. 47 figs. XII, 325 pp. ISBN 3-540-43261-2

Vol. 270: **Beutler, Bruce; Wagner, Hermann (Eds.):** Toll-Like Receptor Family Members and Their Ligands. 2002. 31 figs. X, 192 pp. ISBN 3-540-43560-3

Vol. 271: **Koehler, Theresa M. (Ed.):** Anthrax. 2002. 14 figs. X, 169 pp. ISBN 3-540-43497-6

Vol. 272: **Doerfler, Walter; Böhm, Petra (Eds.):** Adenoviruses: Model and Vectors in Virus-Host Interactions. Virion and Structure, Viral Replication, Host Cell Interactions. 2003. 63 figs., approx. 280 pp. ISBN 3-540-00154-9

Vol. 273: **Doerfler, Walter; Böhm, Petra (Eds.):** Adenoviruses: Model and Vectors in VirusHost Interactions. Immune System, Oncogenesis, Gene Therapy. 2004. 35 figs., approx. 280 pp. ISBN 3-540-06851-1

Vol. 274: **Workman, Jerry L. (Ed.):** Protein Complexes that Modify Chromatin. 2003. 38 figs., XII, 296 pp. ISBN 3-540-44208-1

Vol. 275: **Fan, Hung (Ed.):** Jaagsiekte Sheep Retrovirus and Lung Cancer. 2003. 63 figs., XII, 252 pp. ISBN 3-540-44096-3

Vol. 276: **Steinkasserer, Alexander (Ed.):** Dendritic Cells and Virus Infection. 2003. 24 figs., X, 296 pp. ISBN 3-540-44290-1

Vol. 277: **Rethwilm, Axel (Ed.):** Foamy Viruses. 2003. 40 figs., X, 214 pp. ISBN 3-540-44388-6

Vol. 278: **Salomon, Daniel R.; Wilson, Carolyn (Eds.):** Xenotransplantation. 2003. 22 figs., IX, 254 pp. ISBN 3-540-00210-3

Vol. 279: **Thomas, George; Sabatini, David; Hall, Michael N. (Eds.):** TOR. 2004. 49 figs., X, 364 pp. ISBN 3-540-00534X

Vol. 280: **Heber-Katz, Ellen (Ed.):** Regeneration: Stem Cells and Beyond. 2004. 42 figs., XII, 194 pp. ISBN 3-540-02238-4

Vol. 281: **Young, John A. T. (Ed.):** Cellular Factors Involved in Early Steps of Retroviral Replication. 2003. 21 figs., IX, 240 pp. ISBN 3-540-00844-6

Vol. 282: **Stenmark, Harald (Ed.):** Phosphoinositides in Subcellular Targeting and Enzyme Activation. 2003. 20 figs., X, 210 pp. ISBN 3-540-00950-7

Vol. 283: **Kawaoka, Yoshihiro (Ed.):** Biology of Negative Strand RNA Viruses: The Power of Reverse Genetics. 2004. 24 figs., IX, 350 pp. ISBN 3-540-40661-1

Vol. 284: **Harris, David (Ed.):** Mad Cow Disease and Related Spongiform Encephalopathies. 2004. 34 figs., IX, 219 pp. ISBN 3-540-20107-6

Vol. 285: **Marsh, Mark (Ed.):** Membrane Trafficking in Viral Replication. 2004. 19 figs., IX, 259 pp. ISBN 3-540-21430-5

Vol. 286: **Madshus, Inger H. (Ed.):** Signalling from Internalized Growth Factor Receptors. 2004. 19 figs., IX, 187 pp. ISBN 3-540-21038-5

Vol. 287: **Enjuanes, Luis (Ed.):** Coronavirus Replication and Reverse Genetics. 2005. 49 figs., XI, 257 pp. ISBN 3-540-21494-1

Vol. 288: **Mahy, Brain W. J. (Ed.):** Foot-and-Mouth-Disease Virus. 2005. 16 figs., IX, 178 pp. ISBN 3-540-22419X

Vol. 289: **Griffin, Diane E. (Ed.):** Role of Apoptosis in Infection. 2005. 40 figs., IX, 294 pp. ISBN 3-540-23006-8

Vol. 290: **Singh, Harinder; Grosschedl, Rudolf (Eds.):** Molecular Analysis of B Lymphocyte Development and Activation. 2005. 28 figs., XI, 255 pp. ISBN 3-540-23090-4

Vol. 291: **Boquet, Patrice; Lemichez Emmanuel (Eds.)** Bacterial Virulence Factors and Rho GTPases. 2005. 28 figs., IX, 196 pp. ISBN 3-540-23865-4

Vol. 292: **Fu, Zhen F (Ed.):** The World of Rhabdoviruses. 2005. 27 figs., X, 210 pp. ISBN 3-540-24011-X

Vol. 293: **Kyewski, Bruno; Suri-Payer, Elisabeth (Eds.):** CD4+CD25+ Regulatory T Cells: Origin, Function and Therapeutic Potential. 2005. 22 figs., XII, 332 pp. ISBN 3-540-24444-1

Vol. 294: **Caligaris-Cappio, Federico, Dalla Favera, Ricardo (Eds.):** Chronic Lymphocytic Leukemia. 2005. 25 figs., VIII, 187 pp. ISBN 3-540-25279-7

Vol. 295: **Sullivan, David J.; Krishna Sanjeew (Eds.):** Malaria: Drugs, Disease and Post-genomic Biology. 2005. 40 figs., XI, 446 pp. ISBN 3-540-25363-7

Vol. 296: **Oldstone, Michael B. A. (Ed.):** Molecular Mimicry: Infection Induced Autoimmune Disease. 2005. 28 figs., VIII, 167 pp. ISBN 3-540-25597-4

Vol. 297: **Langhorne, Jean (Ed.):** Immunology and Immunopathogenesis of Malaria. 2005. 8 figs., XII, 236 pp. ISBN 3-540-25718-7

Vol. 298: **Vivier, Eric; Colonna, Marco (Eds.):** Immunobiology of Natural Killer Cell Receptors. 2005. 27 figs., VIII, 286 pp. ISBN 3-540-26083-8

Vol. 299: **Domingo, Esteban (Ed.):** Quasispecies: Concept and Implications. 2006. 44 figs., XII, 401 pp. ISBN 3-540-26395-0

Vol. 300: **Wiertz, Emmanuel J.H.J.; Kikkert, Marjolein (Eds.):** Dislocation and Degradation of Proteins from the Endoplasmic Reticulum. 2006. 19 figs., VIII, 168 pp. ISBN 3-540-28006-5

Vol. 301: **Doerfler, Walter; Böhm, Petra (Eds.):** DNA Methylation: Basic Mechanisms. 2006. 24 figs., VIII, 324 pp. ISBN 3-540-29114-8

Vol. 302: **Robert N. Eisenman (Ed.):** The Myc/Max/Mad Transcription Factor Network. 2006. 28 figs. XII, 278 pp. ISBN 3-540-23968-5